THE DIY CARDIOVASCULAR CURE

A COMPREHENSIVE PROGRAM TO REVERSE ATHEROSCLEROSIS

G. A. MOHR, PhD

G. A. Mohr, PhD

THE DIY CARDIOVASCULAR CURE
A COMPREHENSIVE PROGRAM
TO REVERSE ATHEROSCLEROSIS

Transworld Research and Innovation (TRI)
9 Hampstead Drive
Hoppers Crossing VIC 3029
AUSTRALIA

ALSO BY G. A. MOHR

A Microcomputer Introduction to the Finite Element Method
A Treatise on the Finite Element Method
Finite Elements for Solids, Fluids, and Optimization
The MBS: A Course in Management Science
Finite Elements and Optimization for Modern Management
Natural Finite Elements Using Basis Transformation
The Pretentious Persuaders,
A Brief History & Science of Mass Persuasion

Curing Cancer & Heart Disease,
Proven Ways to Combat Aging, Atherosclerosis & Cancer

The Variant Virus, Introducing Secret Agent Simon Sinclair
The Doomsday Calculation, The End Of The Human Race
The War of the Sexes, Women Are Getting On Top
Heart Disease, Cancer, & Ageing:
Proven Neutraceutical & Lifestyle Solutions

2045: A Remote Town Survives Global Holocaust
The History & Psychology of Human Conflict
Elementary Thinking for the 21st Century
The 8-Week+ Program to Reverse Cardiovascular Disease
The Scientific MBA
Mohr's Law of Hierarchies

ALSO WITH R.S. MOHR/RICHARD SINCLAIR & P.E. MOHR/EDWIN FEAR

The Evolving Universe: Relativity, Redshift and Life from Space
World Religions: The History, Psychology, Issues & Truth
World War 3, When & How Will It End?
The Brainwashed, From Consumer Zombies to Islamic Jihad
Human Intelligence, Learning & Behaviour
The Psychology of Hope
New Theories of The Universe, Evolution, and Relativity
The Population Explosion

Table of Contents

PREFACE

Effective health care depends upon self care . . .
Ivan Illich, *Medical Nemesis* (1975).

Since my teens I have had an interest in medical matters. I once spent part of my school holidays helping my mother, a lecturer in pharmacy, and in my penultimate school year I chose Jürgen Thorwald's *The Century of the Surgeon* as a prize which discusses the great advances in medicine that came with the introduction of antiseptics and anaesthetics.

I was just 28 when I first had mild heart pains and what may have been a TIA (mild stroke). The next year I went Cambridge to do my PhD working on the *Finite Element Method* (FEM) which can be used to model the effects of obstructions in blood vessel networks (Mohr, 2012b, 2013).

I had quite severe heart pains after a friendly game of tennis in Cambridge in 1976, not realizing then that I'd had a mild heart attack.

In following years I continued to experience chest pains and other symptoms of vascular problems, for example more serious TIAs in 1981 and 1984. There were even slight after-effects for a few months after the 1981 episode, namely numbness in my left foot and to the left of my top lip, symptoms typical of mild strokes (Newcombe, 2005).

These episodes were few and far between, however, until I was in my mid 50s when the chest pains became regular and I had attacks of stasis dermatitis and ulceration as a result of peripheral vascular disease. I also began to experience pain in my neck which I later realized was caused by a clogged left carotid artery, these becoming quite acute a couple of years later towards the end of 30 to 60 minute road bike rides for exercise.

A decade ago my look-alike eldest brother had heart bypass and heart valve replacement operations and recently one of his sons had the same operations. My eldest brother died recently of a stroke.

Like my eldest brother, I had grown up on a diet with too much saturated fat and had had through adult life somewhat stressful work habits. Worse still, I had been a heavy smoker until nearly 50, perhaps the reason for heart symptoms and TIAs at an early age.

I belatedly gave up smoking on January 1st 1995 at age almost 49.

Then I began to dabble in vitamin tablets and think about *atherosclerosis*. Over time I collected a number of books on diet, taking great notice of reports of niacin's ability to improve cholesterol levels, and Raymond Kurzweil's book *The 10% Solution for a Healthy Life* which shows that restricting dietary fat intake to 10% of total calorie intake, in conjunction with exercise, dramatically improves cholesterol levels and greatly reduces statistical risk of both heart disease and cancer.

Then I wrote the draft of a book on heart disease and cancer in 2003. This was greatly expanded and published in 2012 (Mohr, 2012b). After further work a second edition of this was published (Mohr, 2013), followed by a book on reversing heart disease (Mohr, 2015).

The present book refines the latter book's treatment of heart disease to provide a more concise and easy to follow program.

I hope the book will help people tackle the difficult problems of atherosclerosis using well-known supplements such as niacin, lecithin, garlic, fish oil, seed oils, and key vitamins, minerals and amino acids, along with promising less well-known ones such as the tocotrienol forms of vitamin E, punicalagins in pomegranate juice, and procyanidins in red wine.

Note that the program in Chapter 20 of this book can be described as a startup program because 8 weeks is sufficient to normalize one's cholesterol levels, as demonstrated in *The 8-Week Cholesterol Cure* (Kowalski, 1987). This period is the sort of period it takes to quit smoking and be reasonably confident of having done so for keeps.

Then, as detailed in Chapter 21 the diet, supplements and exercise programs of this book should be continued for two years to achieve significant regression of atherosclerosis, as demonstrated by the Ornish Lifestyle Heart Trial at UCLA (Ornish, 1996) and the Heidelberg Regression study (Superko, 2004).

Finally, thanks to Richard Mohr and Peter Mohr for lending their support as coauthors of several recent books.

Dr Geoff Mohr (PhD), 2018

Disclaimer

A great deal of international research has shown that many of the recommendations given in this book concerning diet, supplements and exercise do reduce cholesterol levels and reduce risk of vascular disease and cancer. Remember, however, that a considerable effort is needed to compile a diet and exercise program that really works and works well for you.   Generally, people concerned about high blood pressure, for example, make only a token effort by cutting down on one or two things such as salt in their diet and doing just a little walking occasionally.

It takes a great deal more effort than this to reduce BP or cholesterol levels *naturally* and this effort must be sustained to *reverse* the damage caused by cholesterol. The reward is that such efforts will also reduce heart attack, stroke and cancer risk.

Kurzweils "10% solution" fat calories diet has had considerable success in reversing heart disease, often in people for whom all other treatments had failed (Kurzweil, 1993). Niacin, along with several other supplements, is also helpful in tackling heart disease, as championed in Kowalski's *The 8-Week Cholesterol Cure* (1987).

As in some of the case studies mentioned in this book, heart disease can be cured by strict diet, exercise, and stress reduction regimens.

Note that the program in Chapter 20 of this book can be described as a startup program because 8 weeks is sufficient to normalize one's cholesterol levels, as demonstrated in *The 8-Week Cholesterol Cure* (Kowalski, 1987). This period is the sort of period it takes to quit smoking and be reasonably confident of having done so for keeps. Then, as detailed in Chapter 21 the diet, supplements and exercise programs of this book should be continued for two years to achieve significant regression of atherosclerosis, as demonstrated by the Ornish Lifestyle Heart Trial at UCLA (Ornish, 1996) and the Heidelberg Regression study (Superko, 2004).

Finally, note that a physician should always be consulted in the first instance about any health concerns and in serious cases of heart disease prescription drugs such as alpha adrenergic receptor blockers may be required (Griffith, 2013), whilst in 'chronic' cases, pharmacological pain management might be required (Lubkin & Larsen, 2006).

Chapter 1

ATHEROSCLEROSIS

> *It is part of the cure to wish to be cured.*
> Lucius Annaca Seneca, 4? BC - 65AD.

The importance of good circulation

As noted in the Preface, I first had symptoms of atherosclerotic heart disease, namely mild angina, at around the age of thirty, these symptoms increasing in frequency and severity and spreading throughout my body over the next three decades, by which time I had begun in earnest the several years of research that led to this and preceding books on heart disease and cancer (Mohr, 2012 – 2015).

Put loosely, atherosclerosis is clogging of the arteries by fatty deposits, resulting in them becoming anoxic, calcifying and hardening. Partial blockage of the blood vessels increases blood pressure, hardening reducing their ability to expand and exacerbating the situation.

Ultimately, clogged and inflexible coronary arteries are finally blocked by clots, resulting in heart attack, or clots move to and block small blood vessels in the brain, resulting in strokes.

Today, therefore, most of us are aware that we should, for example, largely avoid saturated fat as this a principal cause of atherosclerosis and thence heart disease and stroke, two of the mankind's major killers.

There are four other important reasons to avoid atherosclerosis:

(a) Arterial obstruction reduces oxygen supply to tissues, making them more vulnerable to cancer initiation.

(b) Reduced circulation of both blood and lymph reduces cleansing of tissues, increasing cancer risk.

(c) Unhealthy arteries encourage blood clots which can carry cancer cells to form cancer metastases.

(d) Unhealthy arteries also reduce brain function.

Keeping your arteries healthy, therefore, will keep you younger and fitter and reduce both the risks of heart disease, stroke and cancer.

1

1. ATHEROSCLEROSIS

Discovery of atherosclerosis

Leonardo da Vinci was first to report on what we now call atherosclerosis. On dissecting the corpse of a young child and that of an old man who had died of old age he recorded that the old man's arteries seemed *"desiccated"* (Carey, 1995):

I carried out the autopsy to determine the cause
of such a calm death and discovered that it was the result of
weakness produced by insufficiency of blood and of the artery supplying
the heart and other lower members, which I found
to be all withered, shrunken and desiccated.
The other postmortem was on a child of two years, and here
I discovered the case to be exactly the opposite of the old man.

This 'hardening of the arteries,' once called arteriosclerosis, is caused by fatty deposits called *atheroma* in the arteries and is called *atherosclerosis* (here sometimes abbreviated to AS) because in Greek atheroma means 'porridge' and sclero means 'hard' (Westcott, 2002).

Theories of ASHD

Theories as to the causes of atherosclerotic heart disease (ASHD) have included:

1. **The aging theory** that we develop atherosclerosis (AS) from an early age and it affects us to various degrees later. This is disproved by autopsies finding elderly people without AS while some young people develop severe AS.

2. **The metabolic theory** that improper or imbalanced *lipid metabolism* is the cause of AS and this finds support from:

(a) Many epidemiological studies finding a correlation between elevated cholesterol levels and ASHD. For example, total cholesterol (TC) levels in the USA are as high as 200 - 250 where ASHD is common, and as low as 100 - 150 in Japan where it is comparatively rare.

(b) Epidemiological studies finding a correlation between high intake of saturated fats and development of ASHD. For example, Japanese people living in Japan have much less ASHD than those living in Hawaii and LA.

3. The stress theory that the stress of 'high tech' societies causes ASHD is supported by the much lesser frequency of ASHD in relatively primitive societies. It was also supported by a study that found the number of artery cells undergoing mitosis in rats with high BP is 10 times that in normotensive rats (Luckman & Sorensen, 1980).

4. The hormone theory that sex hormones play an important role in ASHD. Thanks to oestrogen young women:
(a) Are relatively immune to AS until after the menopause.
(b) Have higher HDL levels, enabling them to cope with higher total cholesterol and fat storage levels in adipose tissue, particularly around the chest and hips for the mothering function.
(c) Have homocysteine levels around 20% lower than those of men.

Thanks to testosterone, men are geared for more action such as hunting and gathering, and defence, and cannot tolerate as high lipid levels. Physically inactive males, however, store fat mainly around the waste and are highly prone to ASHD.

5. The tumour theory that atherosclerotic plaques are initiated by toxic agents or viruses in the same way as some cancer tumours. Some evidence that atheroma might be a benign tumour of the walls of the arteries, perhaps caused by a latent virus, was found by Dr Edward Benditt at Washington University USA (Luckman & Sorensen, 1980).

6. The virus theory. Recently herpes virus infection of arterial smooth muscle cells has been found to increase cholesterol ester accumulation, this being associated with atherosclerosis (Hsu at el., 1995). Because cholesterol accumulations occur where the body suffers some types of damage, for example scarring or tuberculosis lesions, cholesterol present in atheroma might be the result of the body trying to protect itself.

In addition, there are a number of *environmental factors,* including:
1. Diet.
2. Heavy smoking.
3. Emotional stress.
4. Lack of physical exercise.

There are also relatively rare *genetic factors,* for example familial combined hyperlipidemia (FCH), hypolipemia (hypolipoproteinemia), and homocystinuria.

ASHD usually involves two or more of these negative factors (except for oestrogen, which for pre-menopausal women is a positive factor).

Note in passing that cancer nucleation is probably never 'accidental' mutation (DNA copying error) but also caused by a similar collection of factors (but oestrogen is now a negative factor).

ASHD takes many years to develop. When its symptoms become apparent, and often life threatening, immediate measures that will quickly halt its progression may be called for. Unfortunately, such measures often include major surgery and long-term use of expensive medications.

The causes of atherosclerosis

A Russian scientist discovered the main cause accidentally when studying the effects of a high-protein diet on rabbit kidneys by feeding them meat, eggs, and milk. Dissection showed no kidney damage but severe atherosclerosis, leaving the question of whether it was protein or fat responsible. In 1913, another Russian scientist answered this question by producing severe atherosclerosis in rabbits with a high-saturated fat, protein-free diet (Whitaker, 2002).

Saturated fat is not the only villain and dietary trans fats, cholesterol, and sugar are amongst the other culprits, lack of certain essential vitamins and exercise, of course, being amongst other adverse factors.

An up-to-date description of atherosclerosis

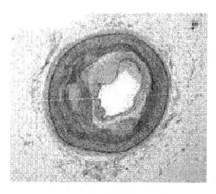

Figure 1.1.
Atherosclerosis
in a coronary artery
(Wikipedia).

Atheroma deposits are caused by oxidation of excess blood lipids, particularly low-density lipoproteins, resulting in fatty spots and streaks inside the arteries. Initially the arteries expand to accommodate them but, with continued deposition, the arteries become clogged.[1]

---

[1] Another mechanism is arteries weakened by lack of nutrients developing small lesions which, in the absence of appropriate nutrients, the body attempts to heal using blood lipids, especially lipoprotein (a).

1. ATHEROSCLEROSIS

The main problem is that when the smooth endothelial lining of an artery is irritated by early lipid deposits an immune response[2] is invoked and white blood cells absorb them, resulting in inflammation that heals in a few weeks (c.f. inflammation around cuts, etc.).

If lipid deposition continues, however, the WBCs become engorged and die, forming fibrous scar-like tissue on the inner surface of the artery (Superko, 2004).

This now rough surface facilitates further lipid deposits which become trapped in connective tissue cells in the inner wall of the artery (the intima) and these enlarged *foam cells* proliferate, resulting in a fatty streak on the inside wall of the artery.

Further lipid deposits penetrate the now softened intima and foam cells begin to burst, setting in motion *fibrosis* as a protective mechanism, so that connective tissue grows through and around the area to seal it off, resulting in a *fibrolipid plaque,* a cyst-like sac filled with lipids,[3] dead cells and other debris which forms between the intima and media (Leonard et al., 1974; Murray, 1977; Luckman & Sorensen, 1980).

These lesions are comparable to adventitious cysts and networks of tiny blood vessels extend into them, continuing a supply of lipids which allows them to continue growing. In part because these networks are incomplete and in part because of the high concentration of fats and cholesterol in them, inner parts of the plaques are starved of blood and nutrients and become necrotic (Heber, 1998).

Initially the artery bulges to accommodate these growths until about 40 to 50% of the cross-sectional area is atherosclerotic material. Then they begin to extend into the lumen.

Initially a plaque is firm and grey or white in colour but as it extends into the lumen and absorbs more fatty materials it softens. Eventually part of the plaque's surface breaks down, forming an ulcer with ragged edges and a base of fibrous scar tissue.

About monthly, plaques have small leaks which are sealed by blood clotting mechanisms to prevent rupture and leakage of necrotic material, further increasing their size (Murray, 1977; Heber, 1998).

---

[2] These lipid deposits may entrap bacteria, encouraging immune response.

[3] Mosby's 1995 Medical Encyclopedia defines atheroma: *an abnormal mass of fat, as in an oil gland (sebaceous), lump (cyst) or in deposits in an artery wall*, and notes that an epidermoid cyst *is filled with oil and dead cells.*

Eventually the inner necrotic material in plaques is replaced by calcified material, hardening them and reducing the likelihood of rupture. Whilst this is, to some extent, a good thing, calcification does indicate a longer history of plaque formation and thence more plaques in one's arteries (Superko, 2004).

Diagnostic scans usually focus upon the largest plaques but usually heart attacks or strokes occur when the thin fibrous cap of a soft, unstable, *vulnerable* plaque causing 30 to 40% blockage ruptures (Heber 1998; Superko, 2004). The released debris attracts clotting factors and inflammatory chemicals in the blood to form a thrombus or clot (Whitaker, 2002). Moving 'downstream' the clot may cause complete blockage at the site of a larger plaque involving 80+% stenosis, or in a smaller artery.

Haemorrhagic strokes occur when a plaque that may have extended into the outer artery layer, the adventitia, ruptures and the weakened artery wall breaks.

Early onset of AS

Early stages of atherosclerosis have been observed in infants at birth, indicating that their mothers' diets had been responsible for such early onset.

In 300 autopsies performed on US soldiers killed in Korea, more than half showed signs of coronary artery damage from plaques. In 100 autopsies carried out on US soldiers killed in Vietnam in 1971, 45% showed medium artery damage and 5% showed severe artery damage. The average age of the soldiers at time of death in both studies was 22 (Leonard et al., 1974).

Rapid progression of AS

In the late 1950s a rhesus monkey was fed a diet with 42% fat calories and 0.02 ounces (about 600 mg) of cholesterol daily. After 2 years it developed *xanthomas* (fatty, fibrous, yellowish plaques in the subcutaneous layer of skin), a result of lipid deposits and thus a sign of atherosclerosis, and after 2.5 years it had a massive and fatal heart attack involving about half of its left heart muscle. Autopsy showed many areas of cell death in the heart and the arteries were filled with plaques, results typical of those for human heart attack victims (Taylor et al., 1963).

The experiment has been repeated many times since, but rhesus monkeys do not normally have heart attacks (Leonard et al., 1974).

Regression of AS

In 1970 Armstrong and his associates fed 30 rhesus monkeys a high fat/cholesterol diet for 18 months, after which 10 were chosen as 'baseline' specimens and examined, showing more than 50% atherosclerotic closure of their coronary arteries (Armstrong et al., 1970).

For the next 40 months 10 monkeys were fed a diet of only 4% fat and no cholesterol, and 10 were given 40% unsaturated fat and no cholesterol. At the end of the test plaques in the monkeys given little fat had been reduced to only 25% of the amount in the baseline monkeys.

The monkeys liberally given unsaturated fat had 50% more plaques than those on the low fat diet, still a substantial reduction from the baseline level (Armstrong et al., 1970).

Other experiments with rhesus monkeys have given similar results (Leonard et al., 1974), such experiments establishing the fact that saturated fat is a major cause of atherosclerosis.

Such results emphasized the link between dietary fat intake and blood cholesterol levels and motivated a number of people to encourage diets with only 10% of their calories from fat, for example Kurzweil (1993).

The genetic picture

Today we have an "epidemic" of obesity in some advanced Western economies. This is a result of *metabolic syndrome* when people consume high GI foods and pile on weight, resulting in much greater risk of diabetes and kidney failure, not to speak of much increased risk of heart disease and cancer (Kurzweil, 1993).

Sadly, this is in part owing to epigenic marks laid down by both parents at the point of conception, a process called metabolic imprinting. Thence if mum &/or dad is obese, the likelihood of the child following suit sooner rather than later is increased.

The message is clear. With the world's human population at least twice what is should be (Mohr, 2012), not only should we be more inclined to have only one or two children, if that, but we should take much greater care to keep our own bodies and minds in good order before doing so.

Conclusion

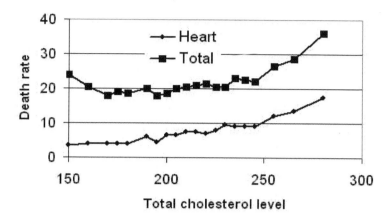

Figure 1.2. Death rates from all causes (upper)
and from heart disease (lower) vs. blood cholesterol level.
Death rate is the age-adjusted six-year death rate
per 1,000 men (Martin et al., 1986).

In the 1940s and 1950s a consequence of primary industry policy of promoting high consumption of beef, fats, and sugar was an epidemic of male heart disease (Gardner, 1992). Since that time awareness of the important role cholesterol plays in heart disease has grown.

Figure 1.2 clearly shows that higher cholesterol levels increase death rates, particularly from heart disease. The message is clear: reducing total serum cholesterol level below 200 reduces rates of mortality from heart disease and also other causes. By so doing atherosclerosis can be prevented or at least reduced. Indeed, with enough dietary diligence, along with suitable dietary supplements and a comprehensive exercise program, it is often possible to reverse atherosclerotic damage and this is a major purpose of this book.

Some of the measures taken to tackle atherosclerosis, for example minimizing body weight and ensuring a good dietary intake of vitamins and antioxidants, will also reduce aging and the risk of cancer, the other aims of this book.

Chapter 2

THE MOHR FORMULA
FOR HEART DISEASE

> *. Lecithins are found in the liver, nerve tissue, semen, bile, and blood. They are essential for transforming fats in the body.*
> *Deficiency leads to liver and kidney disorders,*
> *high serum cholesterol levels, atherosclerosis, and arteriosclerosis.*
> Mosby's Medical Encyclopedia, 1995.

Lecithin

Commercial lecithin is a mixture of phospholipids (phosphatides) containing principally 13-18% lecithin (phosphatidyl choline), 10-15% cephalin (phosphatidyl ethanolamine), 10-15% phosphatidyl inositol, 5-12% phosphatidic acid, and about 35 percent neutral oil (American Lecithin Company, Oxford CT).

Pure lecithin is white and waxy and darkens when exposed to air. Commercial lecithin, most of which comes from soybean oil, is brown to light yellow and its consistency varies from plastic to liquid. Lecithin is widely used as an emulsifying and wetting agent because it retards oxidation, retains moisture and disperses globules of fat.

Phospholipids are important constituents of cell membranes and of the membranes of cell components such as mitochondria. They function in the conduction of nerve impulses, in the insulation of nerve cells, in certain enzyme-catalyzed reactions within cells, in blood coagulation, and transport of lipids from the liver to other tissues and organs in mammals.

Phospoholipids have a phosphate group at one polar, electrically charged, hydrophilic end, and one or two fatty acids at the other neutral, hydrophobic end. In cell membranes phospholipids form a two-layer structure, called the lipid bilayer in which hydrophilic groups maintain continuity between the water outside and that inside the cell, and hydrophobic groups dissolve lipid materials, allowing them to enter the cell (Encyclopaedia Britannica, 1999).

A cure for heart disease?

According to Dr Roger Williams, who discovered the B vitamin pantothenic acid, lecithin in the blood: " - - tends to dissolve cholesterol deposits. When there is substantially more lecithin in the blood than cholesterol - a ratio of 1.2 to 1 is said to be favourable - the actual amount of cholesterol can be high without the blood plasma getting milky or showing a tendency to produce fatty deposits" (Williams, 1971).

"As early as 1935 it was shown that experimental heart disease, produced by feeding cholesterol [to laboratory animals], could be prevented by merely giving a small amount of lecithin" (Davis, 1972).

Proof that lecithin prevents atherosclerosis in humans came from a Dutch study of 48 men aged 40 to 60 which found that only those with lecithin content of $\leq$ 34% in their blood fats (half of them) had problems associated with atherosclerosis, the rest with $\geq$ 36% lecithin content in their blood fats were free of atherosclerosis (Murray, 1977).

Murray (1977) notes that some doctors prescribe 4 - 6 tablespoons of lecithin daily to treat atherosclerosis and heart conditions when cholesterol levels are high and then 1 or 2 tablespoons daily to maintain low levels.

That lecithins could regress atherosclerosis was demonstrated in the late 1950s when high blood cholesterol levels and atherosclerosis were induced in rabbits fed a diet high in saturated fats and then half of them injected with phospholipids, clearing most of the atherosclerotic deposits (Friedman, Byers, Rosenman, 1957; Byers, Friedman, 1960).

Similar results continued to appear and in 1975 researchers at Upjohn published definitive research confirming that *"in essence, heart disease could be reduced, if not eradicated, through a simple injection"* of phospholipids (Sears, 1995). Indeed, Sears developed a number of new phospholipid compounds to regress atherosclerosis which were *"too good - they were pulling cholesterol from the atherosclerotic lesions, but they were also pulling cholesterol from the red blood cells,"* killing some of the experimental animals. He was, however, able to use phospholipids to successfully deliver otherwise insoluble cancer drugs (Sears, 1995), and IV phospholipids have since been used successfully in conjunction with an apolipoprotein to regress atherosclerosis.

The Dr Rinse Formula

In 1951, Dr Jacobus Rinse, a chemist then aged 51, was given 10 years to live by his doctors after a heart attack and forced to take up to 2 - 4 nitroglycerin pellets per hour. Six years later he heard that soy lecithin had been found able to dissolve cholesterol in animals with experimentally induced high cholesterol levels, and also that safflower oil could liquefy cholesterol (Fischer, 1993).

Already with a strict diet supplemented with vitamins C and E, he began taking a tablespoon each of lecithin and safflower oil daily with breakfast. In just a few days he felt better, saying: *"My angina pains ceased. My galloping pulse rate[1] decreased slightly, but noticeably. Excellent results began to appear within a few days."*

After 3 months his angina had vanished completely, even after exercise. After a year he was doing heavy outside work, and at age 88 he was in robust health and his now famous Dr Rinse Formula based on lecithin + unsaturated oils rich in omega-6 fatty acids had achieved miraculous cures for countless people with a very wide variety of ailments including heart disease, high and low BP, high cholesterol, hypoglycemia, arthritis, bursitis, phlebitis, peripheral vascular disease, gout, osteoporosis, and eye disorders such as glaucoma (Murray, 1977; Fischer, 1993).

For example:

(a) Elna Groth N.D., an Austrian naturopath wrote: *"I learned of the Dr Rinse Formula and have since used it on many hundreds of my patients suffering health conditions that don't normally respond well to any medication. I have seen the most wonderful results with this mixture of vitamins in such cases as heart disease, angina and other coronary problems. Many of my patients afflicted with arthritis, gout, varicose veins, high cholesterol and even eye disorders, such as glaucoma, have responded favourably"* (Fischer, 1993).

(b) *"A Vermont woman, 70 years of age, had survived blockings in the neck artery and partial paralysis. She began the Rinse regimen and her health improved rapidly. She has had no recurrences, Dr Rinse said. Clinical tests showed that all cholesterol deposits had disappeared"* (Murray, 1977).

---

[1] Either tachycardia (pulse > 140) or arrhythmia (irregular heartbeat).

(c) *"A Dutch internist told Dr Rinse that he prescribed the special breakfast for many of his older patients. Many of them soon resumed their activities, even though they had been invalids for a long time"* (Murray, 1977).

(d) A woman in Iowa wrote: *"The results I have obtained with your formula were startling. In just 16 days my blood pressure dropped noticeably. My angina pains are all but gone. After two months, I could exercise with no pain."* (Fischer, 1993).[2]

The Dr Rinse formula (for a 2-week supply) is (Fischer, 1993):

7 Tbsp (US) lecithin granules
[1 Tbsp US = 0.7 - 0.75 Tbsp UK or 8.4 - 9 gm of lecithin[3]]
6 Tbsp sunflower seeds [the 2 key ingredients (Murray, 1977)]
6 Tbsp raw wheat germ
6 Tbsp debittered brewer's yeast (powder or flakes)
6 tsp bonemeal from a reliable source (powder or tablets)
6 500 mg vitamin C tablets
6 200 IU vitamin E tablets

Seeds are used rather than oil to avoid the considerable damage which processing tends to inflict upon seed oils. A similar formula is given by Murray (1977) but safflower oil is used instead of sunflower seeds and it is recommended that: *"For severe cases of hardening of the arteries the quantity of lecithin should be doubled."*

How it works

Normally, lecithin plays a vital role in dealing with 'fat overloads' so that when a diet high in fat is taken, there is large increase in the production of lecithin. This helps in changing the fat in the blood from large particles to smaller ones. When one has atherosclerosis, however, the levels of lecithin in the blood remain low regardless of the quantity of fat entering the bloodstream, so that fat particles remain too large to be able to pass through the arterial walls and are deposited on or in them.

---

[2] Rapid reduction in angina symptoms in such cases as this is the result of greater emulsification of blood fats, improvement in vascular flexibility, smoothness, and permeability, and improved nutrient delivery to heart muscle.

[3] Microsoft Bookshelf 1996, World Book 1999, Borushek (2006).

Lecithin also helps maintain the surface tension of cell membranes, thus controlling what goes in and out of each cell, allowing nutrients in, or wastes out. Without enough lecithin, cell membranes harden, not allowing enough nutrients in or wastes out, resulting in premature aging of cells. The result is atherosclerosis in the walls of arteries or diminution of nerve impulse and message transmission in nerve and brain cells.

Two papers published in the journal of the American Oil Chemists Society in 1963 and 1974 showed that cholesterol is soluble in the bloodstream when sufficient lecithin is present. Dr Rinse's formula is especially effective because lecithin, in conjunction with omega fatty acids, reduces the melting point of oxidized cholesterol from 300F to 32F, whereas with lecithin alone the reduction is only to 180F (Fischer, 1993).

As Table 2.1 shows, HDL is rich in 'pure' lecithin and sphingomyelin[4], a sphingolipid containing phosphorus which is abundant in nervous tissue, lecithin being the most important phospholipid in HDL's antiatherogenic reverse cholesterol transport role (Tchoua et al, 2009).

Table 2.1. Composition of blood plasma lipoproteins. (Encyclopaedia Britannica, 1999).

	HDL	LDL	VLDL
Lipids, %	37	48	90
Lipid breakdown, %			
Phosphatidyl choline (lecithin) & sphingomyelin	44	24	20
Triglyceride	20	16	56
Cholesterol ester	24	12	8
Cholesterol	6	12	8
Free fatty acid	6	1	1
Protein, %	45	15	10
Water, %	18	37	0
Density, grams/cc	1.13	1.04	0.91
Diameter, m x 10^{-10}	84	185	500
Approx. molecular wt x 10^6	0.3	2	8

LDL, on the other hand, carries 70% of the cholesterol in the blood whilst VLDL carries most of the triglycerides, and it is these lipids that we seek to minimize in tackling atherosclerosis.

---

[4] According to Mosbys Medical Encyclopedia sphingomyelin is also a phospholipid (Mosby Year Book Inc., 1995).

An improved formula

As Table 2.2 shows, a drawback of the Dr Rinse formula is that safflower or sunflower seeds provide only omega-6 oils which are the most easily oxidized fats (Carper, 2000) and which lower blood levels of both LDL and HDL cholesterol (Cooke and Zimmer, 2002).

Table 2.2. Omega oils content of some common food oil sources.

Source	Fat content % (approx.)	Omega content - % of fats	
		Omega-3	Omega-6
Linseed/flaxseed	34	58	14
Pumpkin seed	33	15	42
Soybean	20	9	50
Rapeseed/canola	30	7	30
Walnut	50	5	51
Safflower seed	58	0	75
Sunflower seed	50	0	65
Sesame seed	50	0	54
Peanut	50	0	29
Almond	53	0	17
Macadamia	72	0	10
Olive	20	0	8
Wheat germ	10	0	54
Rice bran	10	0	35

Today, however, we are much more aware of the importance of omega-3 oils which enhance production of NO (the EDRF) and prostacyclin (PGI_2), and reduce production of thromboxane, thus relaxing blood vessels, improving blood flow, reducing thickening of blood vessels, and preventing blood clots. They also reduce LDL but increase HDL, reduce production of free radicals, and reduce blood vessel inflammation and thence arteriosclerosis (Cooke and Zimmer, 2002).

To tackle ASHD 2 rounded tsp (approx. 7.5 grams) of lecithin granules + 2 rounded tsp of linseeds[5] or 2 tsp (approx. 10 ml) of canola oil can easily be blended into the main dinner course, providing a good balance of omega-3 and omega-6 oils. Kibbled linseed may be used to ensure complete digestion/absorption of linseed nutrients.

---

[5] Linseeds are a good source of amygdalin (vitamin B17), a good protection against cancer, if not cure (Mohr, 2013), and in a study of 161 men with prostate cancer linseeds reduced tumour growth (4 Dec. 09, USAtoday.com).

In addition, one or two niacin tablets[6] should also be had.

For more severe cases such as debilitating angina an additional 2 - 4 rounded tsp of lecithin may be had with other meals during the day,[7] perhaps with less or no linseeds or oil to keep fat intake low.

Soybean lecithin is recommended. It has been found that lecithin from a vegetable source such as soybeans is more effective than lecithin from an animal source such as eggs in re-absorbing arterial cholesterol deposits back into the bloodstream, in part because vegetable-derived lecithin's fats are 80% unsaturated, in stark contrast to lecithin from animal sources.

Finally, linseeds are also high in fibre, one third of it being soluble, and they are the richest known source of special fibre compounds called lignans, which are a class of phytoestrogens. Lignans have cholesterol-lowering properties and help combat heart disease.

The doubters

Because 'natural' compounds cannot be patented Sears developed powerful new phospholipids but drug companies were not interested because they could not be taken as a pill (Sears, 1995). Similarly, there have often been attempts by the medical and pharmaceutical industry to ignore and/or discredit 'natural' solutions to major health issues.

An example of prejudice, perhaps, Borushek and Borushek (1981) make a number of statements, here dealt with in turn:

(1) "Extravagant claims have been made for dietary lecithin."

Response: But too many in number by too many well qualified and experienced people to be dismissed lightly, for example: Davis, 1972; Murray, 1977; Jiminez et al., 1990; Buchman et al., 1992; Fischer, 1993; Brook et al., 1996; Wilson et al., 1998. In addition, Internet search for 'lecithin' yields much discussion of the wide variety of benefits of lecithin.

(2) "The body makes lecithin as required."

Response: Additional dietary lecithin has many benefits, for example,

(a) Lower cholesterol and triglyceride levels, and higher HDL levels.

(b) Increased blood vessel elasticity and prevention of plaques.

(c) Improved delivery of nutrients and removal of wastes in the body.

(d) Improved nerve and brain function.

---

[6] Niacin, a popular remedy for poor cholesterol levels, tends to reduce choline levels and lecithin fixes this problem.

[7] Various websites recommend 1 - 3 Tbsp (US) of lecithin daily.

(3) "Less than 10% [lecithin] is absorbed unchanged, and this explains why large amounts of extra lecithin must be taken for any claimed effect to take place."

Response: But greater availability of the component compounds such as choline (Buchman et al, 1992) facilitates greater lecithin synthesis in the body (Murray, 1977) and, perhaps in severe cases, injection could be used as in numerous successful animal studies referred to earlier.

High niacin dosage to reduce cholesterol levels can deplete choline. Additional lecithin in the diet overcomes this problem, lecithin itself also improving blood lipid levels [see 2(a) above].

(4) "There is no difference in the lecithin blood levels of healthy people and those with atherosclerosis."

Response: Untrue: (a) In the January 1958 issue of *Geriatrics* Dr Lester Morrison published his finding that, in 80% of his patients with high serum cholesterol levels, levels were lowered by an average of 41% after taking lecithin for several weeks, reporting that *"lecithin was found to be the most effective cholesterol lowering agent tested."*

(b) There is a strong correlation between high LDL and VLDL levels and low HDL levels and atherosclerosis and, as Table 2.1 shows, higher HDL levels correspond to higher lecithin levels in the blood.

(c) When not properly emulsified fats tend to cause atherosclerosis, blood clots and thrombosis (Brook et al., 1986). Thus research has shown that atherosclerosis can be induced in the laboratory both by increasing dietary cholesterol intake and by decreasing lecithin intake.

That Dr Rinse's formula brought him no income whatsoever (Murray, 1977) also adds credibility to the claims made for it by many grateful users. The bottom line, therefore, is that lecithin may be of considerable benefit in reducing and even reversing atherosclerosis.

As noted earlier, lecithin and the Dr Rinse formula have produced remarkable results for countless people with a wide variety of ailments. Yet another way in which the fat emulsifying action of lecithin is found beneficial is in combating recurrent plugged milk ducts in breastfeeding mothers, in which case a maximum dosage of 4.8 gm is recommended (kellymom.com).

This, indeed, is a clear and visible example of how lecithin might be helpful in preventing and even reversing atherosclerosis.

For decades research has continued to confirm the beneficial effects of lecithin upon lipid levels, for example reduction of triglyceride levels, (Brook et al., 1986), improvement of lipoprotein composition (Jiminez et al., 1990), and lowering of total cholesterol levels without lowering HDL levels (Wilson et al., 1998).

On the many other benefits of lecithin: "Lecithin has several other benefits aside from reducing cholesterol level. It helps rebuild cells and organs that need it. It keeps the organs healthy. Sufficient intake of lecithin can also delay the aging process" (lecithinguide.com).

Vitamins C and E

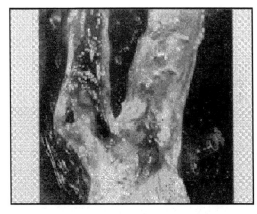

Figure 2.1.
Advanced
atherosclerosis.
[*Atheroma,*
Mosby's Medical
Encyclopedia, 1995].

Lack of vitamin C has been found in victims of coronary thrombosis caused by capillary haemorrhage in plaques (Blumenfeld, 1964), and none at all in brain tissue of some stroke victims[8] (Stone, 1972), leading Stone to suggest that 3 to 5 grams of ascorbic acid daily in spaced doses could prevent heart disease and strokes (Murray, 1977).

The Cambridge Heart Antioxidant Study found that after a first heart attack 400 IU of vitamin E daily halved risk of a second, presumably because it reduces oxidation of LDL cholesterol (McGowan, 1998).

Vitamin C also plays an important role in atherosclerosis insofar as it plays an enzymatic hydroxylation role in the production of procollagen[9] from which all 14 different types of collagen in the body are made, and thence in healthy arteries (Myllyla et al., 1978).

---

[8] "In other words, these people probably had latent scurvy" (Murray, 1977).

[9] Procollagen consists of very strong, twisted, 'ropelike' chains of the non-essential amino acids glycine and proline cross-linked by the essential (not synthesized in the body) amino acid lysine to 'glue' them together.

2. The Mohr Formula for Heart Disease

Animal experiments have shown that lack of vitamin C results in plaque formation, Duguid finding that when vitamin C levels were then restored to normal the plaques disappeared (Duguid, 1946).[10]

Pauling and Rath found that guinea pigs given the equivalent of the human RDI of vitamin C developed plaques in only 5 weeks whereas those given the equivalent of 5 gm vitamin C daily did not (Rath, 2001b).

Willis (1953) found that, in a group of animals with sub-optimal levels of vitamin C, lesions appeared in the lining of the coronary arteries at the points at which they were most stressed by repeated stretching and that it was only after these lesions appeared that plaque began to accumulate.[11]

This is because when there is a shortage of vitamin C arterial walls will develop lesions which then attract dangerous lipoprotein(a) particles. Lp(a) is a small very sticky type of LDL discovered by Berg and Mohr (1963) which is the blood lipid largely responsible for plaque formation.

This is the first stage of plaque formation, that of formation of fatty streaks, the second being the body's attempts to heal the lesion using LDL cholesterol [and particularly Lp(a)], calcium and fibrinogen (the main material in scabs that form over external wounds) if it is unable to make enough collagen owing to a lack of vitamin C.

A study conducted by Willis at two hospitals found that 1500 mg of vitamin C daily for 62-192 days reversed plaques in 60% of patients,[12] whereas they progressed in a control group (Willis et al., 1954, Willis, 1957). This was the first time any treatment had resulted in regression of atherosclerosis in humans.

Other studies in both animals and humans followed, showing that when vitamin C levels are elevated atherosclerotic plaques begin to disappear, Krumdieck and Butterworth (1974) also obtaining reduction of plaque deposits in 60% of patients using vitamin C only (Ellis, 2005).

In the early 1980s, two studies demonstrated that calcium in plaque deposits could be chelated by high doses of vitamin C, transported to the kidneys, and excreted (Geoly & Diamond, 1980; Horsey et al., 1981).

---

[10] Duguid used guinea pigs, which are often used to test the effects of vitamin C deprivation because, like humans, they are one of the few animal species whose bodies do not manufacture vitamin C.

[11] These lesions are an early stage of scurvy (Rath, 2001b).

[12] Spittle (1971) found that such supplementation may raise blood lipid levels temporarily as lipids trapped in artery walls are released (Rath, 2001b).

Another role that vitamin C plays, in conjunction with vitamin E, is that both are required for the synthesis of glycosaminoglycan or GAG (Verlangieri, 1985). GAG is a key ingredient in the 'cement' that holds endothelial cells together so that diet deficiency in C and E leads to arterial deterioration and eventually lesions.

This was demonstrated by inducing atherosclerosis in monkeys by feeding them a vitamin-deficient diet, then giving some of them vitamin E. After 8 months the plaque deposits in the monkeys given vitamin E were reduced from 33% blockage to 8% blockage (Verlangieri & Bush, 1992).

A USC study published in 2000 provided evidence of vitamin C's role in collagen formation, finding that 500 mg vitamin C daily resulted in arteries thickening at 2.5 times the normal rate. Whilst this shows that extra vitamin C may help heal damaged arteries, it suggests a risk of excessive arterial thickening with prolonged dosage at this level.

In the June 2000 issue of Life Extension magazine, however, Dr Robert Cathcart points out that any vitamin C-induced artery thickening "is reversing the thinning that occurs with aging," reminding readers of the reductions in mortality of 45% for men and 35% for women when at least 300 mg of vitamin C is had daily in diet and supplements.

Lysine

Lysine, or epsilon-aminocaproic acid, is an essential amino acid necessary for formation of collagen used in connective tissues.

The 1985 Nobel Prize in Medicine was awarded to Michael S. Brown and Joseph L. Goldstein for discovering that when a lesion occurs in the endothelium of a blood vessel 'Lysine Binding Sites' are exposed to the blood and these bind Lp(a) to the lesion, a number of studies in the late 1980s then confirming that it is, indeed, primarily Lp(a) and not LDL cholesterol that causes clogging of arteries (Ellis, 2005).

Then in 1989 there were 3 important findings on lysine:

(a) Two studies showed that Lp(a) can, not only attach itself to the Lysine Binding Sites of damaged coronary arteries, but is also involved in the deposition of fibrinogen, the second stage of plaque formation (Hajjar et al., 1989; Salonen et al., 1989).

(b) Gonzalez-Gronow et al. (1989) found that lysine binds to the lysine binding sites exposed by the damaged artery, thereby preventing Lp(a) from doing so.

(c) Harpel et al. (1989) discovered that lysine binds to the free-floating Lp(a) in the blood and thereby prevents it from attaching itself to the lysine binding sites of the damaged artery.

Results (b) and (c) show that lysine can prevent plaque formation.

The Pauling Therapy

In 1990 Matthias Rath and Linus Pauling were granted a US Patent (No. 5278189) for the 'Pauling Therapy' for heart disease, namely the use of lysine + vitamin C to inhibit Lp(a) binding to artery walls,[13] and also to release Lp(a) already bound to artery walls, in other words to regress atherosclerosis, referring to lysine as a *"binding inhibitor"* in this context.

Lysine in the blood having been shown to bind to free-floating Lp(a), Rath and Pauling felt that it might also bind to and release already deposited Lp(a). They thought that vitamin C might then enhance release of Lp(a) from plaques *"by dissociating apo(a)[14] from the LDL-like component of Lp(a),"* and also by hydroxylating lysyl residues in artery walls and thus reducing their binding to them (Rath and Pauling, 1991).

Excellent results have been had with this therapy, for example:

(a) A surgeon found after taking 3 gm of both L-lysine monohydrochloride and vitamin C daily for 6 months that her Lp(a) level had dropped to 14 mg/dl, a reduction of 48% (Datessandri, 2001).

(b) A 67 year-old former chemistry Professor taking 6-7 nitroglycerine tablets daily was able to stop taking it altogether after only 3 weeks of taking lysine + vitamin C (Ellis, 2005).

(c) A biochemist with a 30-year history of effort angina and three heart operations was taking beta-receptor and calcium-channel blockers and lovastatin as medication. He also added 6 gm of vitamin C, 60 mg CoQ-10, a multivitamin and mineral tablet, additional vitamins A, E and B-complex, lecithin, and niacin, but still had to take nitroglycerin daily and his angina was still getting worse.

Pauling suggested that he also take 5 gm lysine and after taking 1 rising to 5 gm lysine for just 6 weeks his effort angina had vanished, a result he described as "bordering on the miraculous" (Ellis, 2005).

---

[13] They described Lp(a) as a 'surrogate' for vitamin C and calcium.

[14] In another paper Rath and Pauling documented that the apoprotein (a) part of Lp(a) was just as adhesive as the lipid part (Rath & Pauling, 1991b).

(d) A two-year study of 55 patients aged 44-67 found coronary artery calcification increasing by an average 44% in the first year. Taking 2.7 gm C, B-complex, 600 IU E, 450 mg each of L-lysine and L-proline, 390 mcg folic acid, 30 mg CoQ10, and 450 mg citrus bioflavonoids, decreased the rate of progression in the second year.

In patients with early stage heart disease calcification slowed during the first 6 months of treatment and completely halted or even reversed in the final 6 months (Rath & Niedzwiecki, 1996), suggesting that advanced heart disease might also be halted and perhaps reversed given longer periods of treatment (Rath, 2001b).

Rapid angina reduction in cases (b) and (c) must have been owing to lysine and thence:

(1) Improved levels of NO (nitrous exide), the endothelial-derived relaxation factor (EDRF), and thus vasodilation.[15]

(2) Vitamin C catalyses conversion of lysine into the amino acid carnitine which helps transport fat to the mitochondria for energy production, thus improving heart muscle function.

Studies have found circa 6 gm carnitine daily reduces ischemia, angina and mortality, whilst 1.5-3 gm daily has been found to improve mental function and reduce deterioration in older adults with mild cognitive impairment and Alzheimer's disease.

One Internet version of the Pauling Formula has key ingredients 3 gm vitamin C, 3 gm L-lysine, and 500 mg L-proline, another has only lysine and C, whilst according to Wikipedia the ingredients are vitamin C, lysine and niacin (*Vitamin C megadosage*, Wikepedia 2009).

Lysine is an essential amino acid, that is, it cannot be synthesized in the body, whereas proline[16] is a non-essential amino acid which can be synthesized in the body from glutamic acid. This is why only relatively small amounts of L-proline are included in the Pauling Formula, if any.

When there is sufficient dietary protein, however, it should not be necessary to include L-proline with L-lysine + vitamin C supplementation.

---

[15] Lysine is an essential amino acid needed for proper growth in infants and for nitrogen balance in adults (Mosby's Medical Encyclopedia 1995).

[16] Unimportant amino acid found in many proteins of the body, especially collagen (Mosby's Medical Encyclopedia 1995).

Chelating calcium in arterial plaques

Chelates[17] are compounds consisting of a central metal atom attached to a large organic molecule, called a ligand, in a cyclic or ring structure.

Chelates are more stable than nonchelated compounds of comparable composition and, generally, the more atoms in the chelate ring, the more stable the chelate. Many commercial dyes and such biological substances as chlorophyll and haemoglobin are chelate compounds.

Figure 2.2.
Calcium
ethylenediamine
tetraacetate.

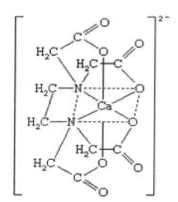

Figure 2.2 shows the chelate calcium ethylenediamine tetraacetate (EDTA).

Chelating agents, particularly salts of EDTA, or ethylenediamine tetra-acetic acid (or edetic acid), are widely used to treat heavy metal poisoning by means of intravenous injection because they bind toxic metal ions more strongly than do organic tissues.

Intravenous EDTA chelation is also used to reduce calcification in atherosclerosis plaques, a process comparable to the way in which vinegar[18] can dissolve eggshells (mostly calcium carbonate).

IV EDTA treatments involve 20 to 50 sessions in which 1 to 3 gm of EDTA is administered, along with vitamin C and other nutrients, taking about 3 hours.

Research has found that the body absorbs only about 5% of orally consumed EDTA and that it takes up to three days for the EDTA to be totally excreted.

---

[17] The word chelate comes from the Greek word *chele* or 'claw.'

[18] Table vinegar is about 4% acetic acid (CH_3COOH).

Thus one would have to take 500mg of EDTA for a month to absorb a similar amount to that given in one low dose IV session. The solution, of course, is that oral dosage must be much greater than IV dosage, and/or much longer term, to have a comparable effect.

As EDTA chelation may deplete vital nutrients, especially minerals, multivitamin and mineral supplements should also be taken.

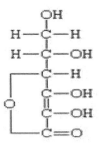

Figure 2.3.

Ascorbic acid (vitamin C).

Figure 2.3 shows the chemical structure of ascorbic acid, one important function of which is to contribute hydroxyl groups (OH) for the hydroxylation reaction required for lysine to link glycine and proline together to form procollagen.

This important role of vitamin C is the basis of Pauling and Rath's vitamin C theory of atherosclerosis. As noted earlier in this chapter, calcium in plaque deposits can also be chelated by high doses of vitamin C.[19]

Indeed, vitamin C tablets are sometimes a combination of ascorbic acid and either calcium, magnesium, potassium or sodium ascorbate,[20] suggesting that it is the ascorbic acid in these which chelates calcium in plaques by becoming calcium ascorbate.

In part chelation reduces arterial calcification because chelating calcium in the bloodstream stimulates production of the hormone parathormone in the parathyroid gland.

This hormone regulates blood calcium levels and when these are low it removes calcium from bones and also the bony structure of calcified arteries to ensure there is sufficient for muscular function.

Pauling and his associates have always advocated megadosage of vitamin C, whether to combat cancer or atherosclerosis.

---

[19] Malic acid, found in winemaking grape varieties such as vitis vinifera, has also been claimed to act as a chelating agent (www.arteryhealthinstitute.com).

[20] Most multivitamin supplements use only ascorbic acid.

Similarly, Cooke and Zimmer (2002) recommend from 3 to 9 grams of L-arginine for endothelial health because only 40 to 50% of the amount ingested reaches the blood vessels, in part because some of it is used for other purposes in the body such as making the neurotransmitter agmatine.

Likewise, dosage of niacin recommended to reduce cholesterol levels is usually about 2 to 3 grams and in the past even higher dosage was sometimes advocated (Kowalsky, 1987).

Finally, so far as the issue of 'megadosage' is concerned, it is encouraging to note that vitamins taken as pills have twice the *bioavailability* of the same vitamins consumed in food (Carper, 2000).

As for dosage of vitamin C required to chelate plaques, assuming that most is used for other purposes such as hydroxylation for procollagen formation, one might expect that dosage of at least 1.5 grams might be required to chelate calcium from arterial plaques, as in the original study by Willis (1957), and in the case of long-standing heart disease perhaps circa 2.5 gm as in Rath & Niedzwiecki's 1996 study.

Vitamins D (circa 5,000 IU)[21] and K, and phytate (from cereal bran) also prevent vascular calcification (VC). In a 10-year study of 4,800 elderly people, 54 mg/day of K2 (RDI = 70 mcg) halved VC and mortality (Geleijnse et al., *J Nutrition* 2004), whilst extremely high dosages of vitamin K reversed VC in rats by 37% in just six weeks (Schurgers et al., *Blood* 109, 2007, 2823-2831).

In addition, keeping the Ca/Mg ratio < or = 3:1 can prevent vascular calcification and populations with 200 - 400 mg magnesium intake have no arterial disease or BP increase with age (Seely S, *IJ Cardiology* 33/2, 1991, 191-198).

Finally, higher HDL levels also correlate with less atherosclerosis.

The Mohr Formula

The results reported for lecithin are remarkable and the list of ailments for which it has been found helpful has grown further, for example:

liver problems, gallbladder disease, dyskinesias, multiple sclerosis, Alzheimer's disease, dementia and bipolar depression.

---

[21] RDI = 400IU. NHMRC UL = 80 mcg = 3200IU.

New benefits of lecithin continue to be found, for example increasing exercise endurance, reducing infertility problems, and improving foetal development. As in the brain and heart, high concentrations of lecithin are found in the prostate gland, suggesting that lecithin may also be of benefit with prostate problems.

As in the Dr Rinse Formula, the use of lecithin in conjunction with omega oils should have the best effect on heart disease because in conjunction they are more effective in dissolving cholesterol.

Lysine + vitamin C also appears to have yielded remarkable results in treating heart disease.

Notably, the reductions in plaque deposits obtained by Krumdiek and Butterworth (1974) using vitamin C alone were reported as involving 'ascorbate-cholesterol-lecithin' interactions, suggesting a combination of two remarkably successful formulas, namely:

(a) Lysine + vitamin C, as in the Pauling Therapy.
(b) Lecithin + linseeds, as in the Dr Rinse Formula.

Some of the most important functions of this combination are:

[1] Lysine competes for free Lp(a) and may also draw it from plaques.

[2] Lysine aids in the production of the EDRF NO and carnitine, which improves fat metabolism and efficiency of oxygen use by heart muscle.
[3] Extra lysine and vitamin C are available for collagen formation for repair of lesions, thus eliminating the need for Lp(a) deposition.

[4] Vitamin C reduces Lp(a) and LDL levels, increases HDL levels, and may be able to bring about release of Lp(a) from plaques.

[5] Vitamin C hyrdoxylates lysyl residues, preventing them from binding to artery walls, and may also chelate calcium from plaques.

[6] Vitamin C increases HDL thereby increasing reverse cholesterol transport (Jacques et al., 1987). It also has anticoagulative properties.

[7] Lecithin lowers LDL levels and emulsifies lipids trapped in plaques, facilitating their release by making cell membranes more permeable.

[8] Lecithin increases capacity for sustained intense exercise which can lower plasma choline levels needed for the neurotransmitter acetylcholine needed for many body functions.

[9] Omega oils increase the solubility of cholesterol and omega-3 oils from fish are particularly beneficial.

[10] Substantial lecithin supplementation might also:

(a) Increase the phospholipid (PL) content of HDL (see Table 2.1), small increases in which "are associated with significant and profound increases in FC [free cholesterol] efflux to serum," thus increasing reverse cholesterol transport [RCT] (Tchoua et al., 2009).

(b) Increase the action of the lecithin-cholesterol acyltransferase (LCAT) enzyme that esterifies free cholesterol[22] for sequestration in the core of plasma HDL and LDL and is important in RCT, including macrophage RCT[23] (Tanigawa et al., 2009). LCAT also reduces the adverse effects of oxidized LDL (Howlader at al., 2001)

As noted in Chapter 13, magnesium is perhaps the most effective treatment for variant angina and it has many other benefits in relation to heart disease, including lowering LDL and TGs, increasing HDL, improving vasodilation, and reducing platelet aggregation.

Thus magnesium supplementation is also included in the Mohr Formula, suggested dosage being circa 500 mg (Lieberman and Bruning [1977] recommend 500-1000 mg for angina).

Linseeds, used in the Mohr Formula to assist absorption of lecithin, contain alpha-linolenic acid (ALA) which the body converts to the same type of omega-3 as found in fish oils. ALA can reduce risk of irregular heartbeat and heart disease, increase metabolic rate, help reduce muscle recovery time after exercise, improve absorption of calcium, and improve condition of the skin, hair and finger and toenails.

Note that, as in the supplement program of Chapter 18, additional supplements should be also had to tackle heart disease, especially fish oil, vitamin E, niacin, and L-arginine.

Chapter 3 summarizes the theory behind the Mohr Formula, also providing a detailed supplement program.

Finally, note that linseeds are a good source of amygdalin (vitamin B17) which helps stop growth of abnormal cells and thence might also be of benefit in reducing atherosclerosis in this way.

---

[22] Phosphatidly choline (lecithin), the most important PL in RCT, contributes the acyl group. It is also "the essential cholesterol-binding component of lipoproteins" (Tchoua et al., 2009).

[23] It is macrophage RCT that regresses atherosclerosis and its rate is a more important antiatherogenic factor than plasma HDL level.

Chapter 3

A UNIFIED THEORY
OF HEART DISEASE

> The findings from the Bogalusa study startled doctors.
> Fifty percent of the children, including some as young as three years old,
> had fatty streaks in their arteries, the first sign of atherosclerosis.
> Fibrous plaques, representing more advanced atherosclerosis, were
> common in ten-year-olds. Seventy percent of young adults had atherosclerosis
> involving both the aorta and the coronary arteries. The evidence was
> incontrovertible: coronary heart disease establishes a foothold in childhood.
> Marc Gillinov & Steven Nissen, *Heart 411* (2012).

Introduction

Chapter 1 gave a brief description of atherosclerosis and Chapter 2 discussed the Dr Rinse formula, Pauling and Rath's 'vitamin C theory' of heart disease, and The 'Mohr Formula' for heart disease briefly. These topics are discussed further and the 'saturated fat', 'homocysteine', and 'vitamin C' theories are combined in a unified theory of heart disease.

Fatty streaks

This, the first stage of development of atherosclerosis, has 3 main causes:

(a) Serum cholesterol levels.

High blood levels of LDL and very sticky lipoprotein (a),[1] and low levels of HDL (which facilitates reverse cholesterol transport), can result in fatty streaks forming on arteries and high consumption of saturated fats and cholesterol contribute to this process, as has been demonstrated in experiments with monkeys (Taylor et al., 1963; Leonard et al., 1974).

---

[1] LDL with apo(a) protein attached. The 'a' stands for adhesive.

Such accumulations of material are more likely at points of lower flow velocity such as at bifurcations and bends, an example of the latter being the circumflex branch of the left coronary artery, other common trouble spots being the carotid arteries and the aorta.

(b) Homocysteine levels

Homocysteine is produced in the blood when the essential amino acid methionine is metabolized, the best sources of methionine being meat, poultry, fish and dairy products.

Homocysteine is normally metabolized and removed from the body. Some people inherit an inability to do this efficiently and generally our ability to deal with homocysteine may decrease as we age. Moreover, high serum homocysteine levels will, of course, compound the problem.

Homocysteine is an "arterial irritant" (Superko, 2004) and some scientists believe that it causes small openings in the cell layer, leading to deterioration of the arterial wall and thence the buildup of arterial plaque (Roizen, 2001).

(c) Vitamin C deficiency and Lp(a).

Vitamin C's most important role is hydroxylation of the reaction by which lysine cross-links chains of proline and glycine to form procollagen.

Anthropoidea, like guinea pigs, are one of the few species that do not synthesize their own vitamin C, no doubt a 'universal' genetic defect in our evolution. Several trials with guinea pigs have shown that vitamin C intake equivalent to the human RDI results in atherosclerosis, whereas increased vitamin C intake eliminates it.

Willis (1953) found that in guinea pigs given insufficient vitamin C arterial lesions formed at points of greatest stress in arteries such as the heart, bifurcations, and bends. Studies in genetically modified mice which do not make their own vitamin C have also shown that lack of vitamin C results in arterial lesions.[2]

These lesions leave exposed lysine and proline binding sites. Without sufficient C available for proper repair very sticky Lp(a), rarely found in species that make their own vitamin C, attaches to these binding sites to form a makeshift patch.

---

[2] Nobuyo Maeda et al., Aortic wall damage in mice unable to synthesize ascorbic acid, PNAS 97/2 (Jan 2000) 841-846.

This is Pauling & Rath's "unified theory" of heart disease which helps complete the picture by providing another mechanism by which fatty streaks develop, few fatty deposits involving LDL alone without Lp(a).[3]

The arterial lesions resulting from lack of vitamin C are an early stage of scurvy, one not suffered by primitive man whose diet contained circa 500 mg vitamin C daily, and it is mitigated by a temporary 'patch-up' process involving Lp(a), an especially sticky form of LDL-C apparently designed for the task.

Formation of plaques

This is the second stage of atherosclerosis. Being very sticky, fatty streaks on the inside of the intima attract LDL, especially Lp(a), VLDL, small dense LDL and oxidized LDL, and perhaps other substances such as insoluble saturated fat, especially if these are present in the blood in high concentrations.

These 'foreign' substances[4] permeate into the artery wall and stimulate immune response and white blood cells invade, gobbling up some of the foreign material.

Bacteria may also be trapped in fatty streaks, providing a major impetus to immune response, and this is the reason for the strong link between periodontitis and heart disease.

As further oxyLDL etc. is deposited the WBC's become engorged (when they are termed foam cells) and die and a cyst-like lesion or fibro-lipid plaque develops, filled with lipids (including intact Lp(a) and oxyLDL), dead WBCs, pus, fibrin and other debris, and covered by a fibrous cap.

This plaque gradually grows and invades the media, causing calcium deposits to form to protect against leakage and aneurysm.[5] As the plaque grows the artery bulges to accommodate it, sometimes doubling or tripling in diameter. Eventually the plaque expands inside the artery, narrowing the lumen.

---

[3] "Lipoprotein-a is the predominant risk factor contributing to the progression of atherosclerotic lesions in man," Matthias Rath, *Reducing the risk of cardiovascular disease with nutritional supplements*, article posted on the Internet.

[4] Lp(a) is not 'foreign' and generally remains intact within plaques.

[5] Arteries thin as we age and, independent of AS calcification (in subdomains of plaques), Mönckeberg's sclerosis or medial calcification occurs to compensate, a process extra vitamin C might prevent. Notably, medial calcification does not occur in coronary arteries.

Note: It is over 'vulnerable' 20-50% blockage (of lumen) plaques that flow velocities and viscous shear (a result of the usual 'zero-max at centre' velocity gradient in pipes) are high enough to contribute to rupture and clot formation and release, resulting in blockage at circa 80+% obstructive plaques or in relatively minor blood vessels downstream. In addition, fibrinogen in the blood is used to form fibrin to help heal ruptured 'culprit' plaques, further enlarging them.[6]

Reversing atherosclerosis

Trials in monkeys in which atherosclerosis was induced by diet high in fats and cholesterol have shown that diet with only unsaturated fat reverses atherosclerosis, more so if total dietary fat intake is also very low (Armstrong et al., 1970).[7]

Animal studies have found that 3-3.5% lecithin dosage prevents atherosclerosis (Wilson et al., *Atherosclerosis* 140(1), Sep. 1998, 147-53) and also reverses it (Hunt & Duncan, *Br J Exp Pathol.* 66(1), Feb. 1985, 35-46).

This dosage is comparable to that of 4-6 Tbsp reportedly advocated by some doctors to reduce cholesterol levels (Murray, 1977). To achieve the somewhat legendary reduction in angina that Dr Rinse originally did in 1957, therefore, this level of dosage will be required.

Several trials with guinea pigs with atherosclerosis induced by low vitamin C intake have shown that increasing vitamin C intake reverses atherosclerosis and repairs damaged arteries (Duguid, 1946; Rath, 2001b).

Additional supplies of essential amino acid lysine may also help in the repair process, this being the basis of the 'Pauling Therapy' in which large amounts of both vitamin C and lysine increase production of carnitine and thus improve muscle function (by improving flow of fats to the mitochondria) and thence reduce angina.

Lysine prevents atherosclerosis by attaching to exposed lysine binding sites in damaged arteries (so that Lp(a) doesn't). It also attaches to and 'neutralizes' Lp(a) in the blood, and may even pull Lp(a) out from plaques (Gonzalez-Gronow et al., 1989; Harpel et al., 1989; Ellis, 2005).

---

[6] Plentiful vitamin C may help heal such ruptured plaques more properly.

[7] In humans only low fat intake can be relied upon to reverse AS (Leonard et al., 1974).

Human trials such as the Ornish Lifestyle Heart Trial showed that restriction to 10% fat calories intake, along with stress-reduction, regressed AS and the Heidelberg Regression Study showed that sufficient exercise can also regress AS.

The Pauling therapy (C + lysine) addresses only the vitamin C deficiency part of the 'unified' theory of heart disease presented here. Thus, though often effective, there are many cases where it proves of little help (www.paulingtherapy.com), probably because serum cholesterol levels have not been improved sufficiently.[8]

The Dr Rinse and Pauling Formulas

In the classical case of Dr Rinse himself, high pulse rate from arrhythmia and effort angina (EA) were relieved by his now famous formula, the key ingredients of which were a tablespoon each of soy lecithin and safflower oil.

Lecithin improves vascular flexibility and heart muscle function by facilitating transport of nutrients and wastes across cell membranes.

In the case of Pauling's 'first patient' to whom 5 gm lysine daily[9] was suggested (case (c) in Sec. 13.9), the problem was also effort angina.

Reduction of blood blow by atheroma reduces carnitine supply to heart muscle where it helps transport fat to the mitochondria for energy production.[10]

Additional lysine and vitamin C are used in part to produce more carnitine[11] which thus improves heart muscle function.[12]

Thus in one study 2 gm carnitine reduced symptoms in CVD patients and in another 6 gm carnitine prevented angina (Cooke & Zimmer, 2002).

---

[8] Pauling therapy failed to lower Lp(a) levels in a UK trial involving 200 men (Ellis, 2005).

[9] Increasing to 6 gm lysine allowed him more intense exercise.

[10] Generally muscles use glucose for energy but heart muscle uses fats for more than 50% of its energy.

[11] Methionine, niacin, B6, and magnesium are also required to produce carnitine.

[12] A major cause of heart disease is that, when fatty acids remain in cardiac cells and tissues because of a lack of carnitine to transport them to the mitochondria, they develop oxidative derivatives which severely damage heart muscle cells. Direct or indirect carnitine supplementation can reverse this damage and prevent heart attacks.

3. The Mohr Formula for Heart Disease

Given time, substantial dosage of vitamin C also:

(a) Reduces Lp(a) and LDL, also increasing HDL levels.

(b) Improves arterial dilation and reduces BP.

(c) Reduces plaques in size (Willis, 1954, 1957).

(d) Chelates calcium from arterial deposits (Geoly & Diamond, 1980; Horsey et al., 1981).

The Mohr Formula

This combines several synergistic supplements:

(1) Lecithin + linseeds (an improved Dr Rinse formula).

(2) C + lysine, the key ingredients of the Pauling formula.

(3) Niacin, used in several trials alone or with statins to reverse atherosclerosis.

(4) Fish oil, one trial using 6 gm/day for 3 months + 3 gm/day for 21 months to reverse AS.

(5) L-arginine to promote nitric oxide (NO), the endothelial-derived relaxation factor.

(6) Vitamin E which has been found to help reverse atherosclerosis, along with other antioxidants including selenium.

(7) B-complex to normalize homocysteine levels.

(8) Magnesium for heart rhythm, vasodilation & variant/stress angina, along with other minerals including calcium and chromium.

(9) 150-300 mg aspirin daily.

(10) A comprehensive multivitamin and mineral supplement.

The following table (Table 3.1) summarizes the synergistic effects of the key supplements of the Mohr Formula for heart disease.

Here most supplements improve vasodilation to help deal with problems of (mental) stress angina (SA) and thence adrenalin-induced vasoconstriction.

Table 3.1. Effects of key supplements of the Mohr Formula.

	Vaso-dilation	Chol. level	Oxidation	Inflamm-ation.	Fat transport	Clotting
Lecithin & linseeds		<		<	>	<
Vitamin C & lysine	>, NO protected	<	<		>	
Niacin	>, via PGI$_2$	<		<	>	
Fish oil	>, via PGI$_2$	<		<		<
L-arginine	>, gives NO					
Vitamin E	>, via PGI$_2$		<			<
Mg	>	<		<		<

Short term (12 - 24w) dosage of C and lysine in the Mohr Formula is at similar levels to those of the Pauling Formula. For the longer term dosage is reduced. For vitamin C, 1500 mg (as in Willis' classical 1954 study[13]), along with sound low-fat diet, reduction of cholesterol levels, and exercise, should be sufficient to reverse atherosclerosis, given time, heavily calcified 'old' plaques taking much longer to reduce in size than newer, smaller and 'softer' ones. Short-term (3 - 6 months) and long-term Mohr Formula dosages (gm daily) are shown in Table 3.2.

Table 3.2. Short-term (ST) & long-term (LT) Mohr Formula dosages (gm, except for vitamin E which is IU)

	Lec.+ linseed	C	Lysine	Niacin	Fish oil	Argin-ine	E	Mg
ST EA dose	7.5 + 7.5	5 - 7	5 - 6	0.1 - 0.2	1	0	500	0.2
ST SA dose	7.5 + 7.5	2	1	0.6 - 1.0	3 - 6	3 - 6	500 - 1000	0.5
LT dose	7.5 + 7.5	1.5 - 2	0.5 - 1	0.1 - 0.2	1	0	500	0.3 - 0.5

---

[13] Willis GC, Light AW, Gow WS, Serial arteriography in atherosclerosis, Canadian MA J vol. 71, Dec 1954.

Here alternative short-term dosage regimes are suggested for exercise-related 'effort angina' (EA), and mental/emotional 'stress angina' (SA), the latter being better for protecting against strokes.

If in doubt both the EA and SA short-term dosage regimens can be tried. Alternatively, the ST EA and SA dosages can be combined, taking whichever is the greater of the dosages in rows 2 and 3 of Table 3.2.

Finally note that:

(a) One study found that E + C + selenium supplementation reduced niacin's HDL raising effects but moderately high vitamin C intake may compensate for this.

(b) High-dose niacin may raise homocysteine levels but B-complex supplements are used normalize these.

(c) A study conducted in Leipzig and published in the American Journal of Cardiology found exercise as effective as taking arginine in increasing vasodilation, a combination of the two increasing vasodilation a further 50%.

A little red wine

Some studies have found low to moderate alcohol consumption to reduce overall disease mortality rates. Even low levels of consumption, however, may increase risk of some cancers, especially those involving the top of the digestive tract.

In contrast, moderate consumption of wine, particularly red wine, does reduce risk of heart attack and stroke.

This is because of the antioxidants in wine, particularly the procyanidins in red wine (Corder, 2007), and also the vasodilatory and anticoagulant effects of alcohol.

Table 3.3 is an adaptation of that given in Appendix A5 of the current Australian NHMRC guidelines (NHMRC, 2009b) and is based on a meta-analysis by Corrao et al. (1999).

Where two rows of figures are given, the first is for men and the second for women. When only one row is given there is no significant risk difference between men and women.

The data shows increased disease risk for all levels of alcohol consumption except for ischaemic heart disease and stroke.

Table 3.3. Relative disease risks vs alcohol consumption.

Disease	Relative risks for 1-10 standard drinks daily									
	1	2	3	4	5	6	7	8	9	10
Lip, oral & pharyngeal cancer	1.31	1.67	2.08	2.53	3.02	3.53	4.06	4.58	5.09	5.57
	1.33	1.72	2.18	2.69	3.26	3.88	4.52	5.19	5.85	6.51
Oesophageal cancer	1.17	1.37	1.61	1.88	2.19	2.55	2.95	3.42	3.94	4.52
Liver cancer	1.08	1.15	1.23	1.31	1.40	1.48	1.56	1.65	1.73	1.81
Breast cancer	1.08	1.17	1.26	1.36	1.47	1.58	1.71	1.85	1.99	2.15
Hypertensive diseases	1.15	1.33	1.53	1.77	2.04	2.35	2.71	3.12	3.60	4.15
Ischaemic heart disease	-	-	-	-	-	-	-	1.01	1.03	1.13
Ischaemic stroke	-	-	-	1.12	1.40	1.73	2.04	2.21	2.12	1.72
Haemorrhagic stroke	1.16	1.35	1.57	1.82	2.12	2.46	2.86	3.32	3.86	4.48
Cirrhosis of the liver	1.21	1.45	1.72	2.02	2.35	2.71	3.10	3.51	3.94	4.38
	1.32	1.73	2.25	2.89	3.68	4.64	5.80	7.17	8.80	10.69

As might be expected, higher levels of consumption pose extremely high risk of cirrhosis of the liver, very high risk of cancers at the top of the digestive tract, and very high risk of hypertensive disease and haemorrhagic stroke.

The analysis only considered risk increase, however, so no risk figures are shown for congestive heart disease for 7 or less SD, or for congestive stroke for 3 or less SD.

This latter figure is suggestive of a safe level of consumption for people concerned only with congestive vascular disease.

Indeed the 15-year study by Serge Renaud in France did find that, amongst 34,000 Frenchmen, 75% of whom drank red wine, 2-3 glasses daily cut death rate by 30%, risk of heart disease by 35%, and risk of cancer by 18-24% (Carper, 2000).

The Mohr Plan for heart disease, therefore, does recommend a couple of glasses of red wine regularly, if not daily, as an additional dietary 'supplement.' Hopefully, this will be consumed in a relaxing manner, conferring additional benefit.

3. The Mohr Formula for Heart Disease

Results?

Angina symptoms resulting from lack of magnesium and/or carnitine may be reduced in days. In as little as 6-8 weeks, as blood cholesterol and sugar levels are improved, AS regression may begin.

In one study, for example, 6 gm of fish oil for 3 months, and then 3 gm for the next 21 months, gave significant regression.

In the Ornish Lifestyle Heart Trial there was slight regression in one year with ultra-low fat diet and stress reduction, whereas the control group experienced significant increase in plaques.

In the Heidelberg Regression Study exercise was largely responsible for significant regression in two years.

With C and lysine as the main supplements, Rath and Niedzwiecki (1996) reversed calcification in patients with early CHD and slowed progression in the rest in two years

Obviously, therefore, combination of low-fat diet, appropriate supplements, exercise, and stress reduction can be expected to regress atherosclerosis, albeit slowly but perhaps a good deal more quickly than it developed – see the following classical results.

Classical results obtained by Willis

Results of Willis et al. (1954) in a trial of vitamin C for patients hospitalized with heart disease. TC = total cholesterol level.

Control group

# age	Diagnosis	Time Days	**Change in Plaques**	TC before mg/%	TC after mg/%	Symptom Changes
1/72	Severe PVD	176	**2 >, 2 =**	N/A	N/A	Impending gangrene
2/74	Severe PVD	70	**4 >; multiple =**	332	290	No Change
3/63	Diabetes	70	**No change**	240	278	No Change
4/77	ASHD, diabetes	82	**No change**	216	232	No Change
5/59	Severe PVD	172	**1 >**	N/A	N/A	Required amputation
6/62	Diabetes	192	**No change**	332	287	No change

Comment: No reduction in plaques in the control group.

Results in Group Given Ascorbic Acid (500 mg 3 times daily)

# age	Diagnosis	Time Days	Change in plaques	TC before mg/%	TC after mg/%	Symptom Changes
7/69	Severe ASHD	62	3 >, 2 =	350	262	Died 1 month later pneumonia
8*/59	Severe PVD Amp. left leg	172	2 <	375	360	No change
9/72	PVD, impending gangrene	136	3 <, 3 =	N/A	N/A	< claudication
10*/58	Old myocardial infarction	125	2 >, several =	323	287	No Change
11/56	Diabetes, xanthomatosis angina pectoris	110	7 <, 7 =	312	216,240, 240	Xanthomata softer, < painful, = size
12*/64	High chol., old myocardial infarction	105	6 >, 2 =	560 to 435	485	No change
13/65	Old myocardial inf., cerebral thrombosis	116	5 =	258	255	No Change
14/61	Diabetes, old myocardial inf.	96	1 <, multiple =	255	312	No Change
15*/55	Diabetes	100	1 <, 6 =	221	248	No Change
16/63	Angina pectoris	155	3 <, multiple =	292	390	Angina much less
Notes: * These cases in error each had a period up to 3 weeks without therapy. All others had continuous therapy.						

Comment: Reduction in plaques in cases 8, 9, 11, 14, 15 & 16, i.e. in 60% of those taking C.

Conclusion:

A remarkable result in a relatively short time with an extraordinarily simple and cheap "therapy."

3. The Mohr Formula for Heart Disease

Chapter 4
DIET DO'S AND DON'TS

> - - *increasing the consumption of important vitamins*
> *seems to be more than twice as important in protecting a person*
> *from heart attack than any other factor.*
> Gey et al. (1991) in a paper on the results of a large WHO study.

Calorie counting

Everyone should have a good idea of how many calories from food they input each day. This is easily ascertained by consulting tables of calories for various types of food given in countless books or, better still, obtaining a book such as Alan Borushek's *Calorie Counter* (2014) which has an almost encyclopedic listing of the calorie or kilojoule content of Australian foods. It also includes tables for the carbohydrate, fibre, sodium, calcium, protein, iron, fat and cholesterol contents of most Australian food products.

Often this is the first step in any weight loss program, the next being to estimate what sort of calorie intake will allow you to lose weight at an appreciable rate. This topic is explored in detail in Chapter 6.

An even more important consideration is examining your diet carefully to see where it might be possible to eliminate some of the less healthy foods in your diet and replace them with healthier alternatives.

For well over a decade before the seeds of the program outlined in this book were sown the author, for example, had just about lived on tea, coffee, cigarettes and booze, skipping breakfast and only having a minimal lunch and a 'dog's dinner' single plate for dinner.

Not being able to cook to any significant extent, after a career disaster and marriage breakdown he lived mainly out of tins or on frozen food such as Dim Sims or meat pies and cheap cocktail frankfurters, most of it full of saturated fat, probably the number one diet villain.

4. DIET DO'S AND DON'TS

Table 4.1. Energy content of some common foods.

Food	calories	kJ
Full cream milk, 200 ml *	134	560
Bottled orange juice, 200 ml *	75	314
Wheat biscuits, two *	100	418
Fried eggs, 2 large 53 gm	200	836
- with 2 small slices bacon	300	1254
Meat pie, 170 gm *	400	1672
Hot dog *	400	1672
Big Mac	575	2404
Ham & salad sandwich	330	1379
200 ml cola drink *	85	355
Baked beans in tomato sauce, 440 gm * can *	400	1672
1/4 large frozen pizza, 125 gm	275	1150
4 fried fish fingers	280	1170
deep fried French fries, 100 gm	320	1338
2 chocolate biscuits	192	803
4 cans 5% alcohol beer *	565	2362
2 glasses (120 ml) dry white wine	150	627
Total of * items	2159	9025

Table 4.1 gives just a few examples of the calorie content of some common foods. If we choose the * items from the list as a day's intake this yields a daily intake of 2159 calories.

The right amount for a 36 to 55 year old male weighing 70 kilos (the right weight if he is 5'10" and of medium build) is 2480 calories if his occupation is sedentary (Borushek, 2014).

The right amount for a woman of the same weight and low level of physical activity is 2050 calories, taken to be less because she supposedly has a larger proportion of fat and less muscle.

Thus the * total of 2159 calories obtained from Table 4.1 is rather low for a 70 kg man and perhaps he would make up the shortfall by having fat laden fast or snack foods, or a 'few' beers, as often as not overdoing it somewhat from the calorie point of view at least.

In the example * but none too good day's diet picked out in Table 4.1 the full cream milk, the meat pie and hot dog, and the cola, are none too good but the baked beans are, in fact, quite healthy except for the fact that, like most canned foods, they are very high in salt.

To get some idea of what is healthy and what is not it is helpful to start by considering the four basic food groups.

The food groups

There are four basic food groups (Consumer Guide, 1979):

1) **Bread and cereals**

Bread, rice and pasta. Four servings a day are recommended.
Three times a day, however, should suffice.

2) **Fruits and vegetables**

The yellow-orange-red coloured fruits are particularly desirable, for example carrots and tomatoes.
Green leafy vegetables are particularly desirable.
Five servings of vegetables and three of fruits are recommended daily and this can include fruit and vegetable juice.

3) **Meat & alternatives**

Lean red meat is reasonably healthy but still quite high in fat.
Avoid 'mystery bags' (sausages, meat pies and hamburgers).
Fish is generally preferable to meat, especially as it contains very healthy omega-3 oils which help lower cholesterol levels.

4) **Milk and dairy products**

Should be avoided except for low fat milk or preferably skim milk which has the same content of desirable calcium. A little yogurt is a possible exception as it has some health benefits.

An additional 'fifth group' can be added, that is: fats, rich desserts and confectionery. These have low 'nutrient density' and are sometimes called 'empty calories' because they are high in calories but contribute little or no protein, vitamins or minerals to the diet.

Nevertheless, some oils such as linseed oil are rich in healthy omega-3 fatty acids and therefore healthy.

In summary, a healthy diet is built on wholegrain breads and cereals, fruit and vegetables, fish rather than meat usually, and low fat dairy products such as skim milk.

4. Diet Do's and Don'ts

Good things to add to your diet

[1] Fruits and vegetables

Fruits and vegetables are rich in antioxidants, for example tomatoes and other red coloured fruits and vegetables contain lycopene, a powerful antioxidant. Not surprisingly, therefore, women who eat plenty of fruit and vegetables are 41% less likely to develop lung cancer (*Journal of the American Medical Association* 294, 1493-1504, 2005).

Fruit and vegetables also have plenty of fibre to speed digestion and increase faecal fats, sterols (including cholesterol) and bile acids.[1] This may in part be why a study of nearly 5000 men and women aged from 40 to 59 found that substitution of vegetable protein for animal protein lowers blood pressure (*Archives of Internal Medicine* 166, 79-87, 2006).

Most diet information sources recommend at least two serves of fruit and five servings of vegetables a day, a serving being about 80 grams.

Brassica vegetables such as cauliflower and cabbage reduce risk of cancer in the first part of the large bowel whilst dark yellow vegetables and apples reduce risk of cancer of the end part of the colon (Annema N et al., *J Am Diet Assoc* 111(2011)1479-90).

[2] Fibre

All types of dietary fibre, except lignin, are polysaccharides (i.e., carbohydrates). By definition, dietary fibre is not digested by human enzymes in the small intestine, but soluble fibre may be digested by fermentation in the large intestine. Insoluble fibre may help reduce absorption of fats and thus assist one in losing weight (Eyton, 1982).

High fibre diets also help remove toxins from the body (Plant & Tidey, 2010), and according to research at Harvard University, heart-disease risk drops 20% for every 10 grams of fibre added to our diets (Somer, 2001).

Fruits, vegetables and wholegrain foods are good sources.

[3] Resistant starch

Wholegrain foods such as wholegrain cereals, wholemeal bread, baked beans and pasta are high in resistant starch. A paper published in *Nutrition & Metabolism* in 2004 (cited in *The Weekend Australian,* 23-24th July 2005) reported that resistant starch helps us burn more fat. In a small trial 12 people had 5.4 per cent of their dietary carbohydrate replaced by resistant starch, increasing metabolization of fat by 23 per cent.

---

[1] Bile acids assist in breakdown and absorption of fats.

[4] Fish

Fish is a good source of protein and has much less saturated fat than red meat. Fish oils also contain the omega-3 fatty acids DHA (docosahexaenoic acid) and EPA (eicosapentaenoic acid) which help reduce heart disease, so much so that heart disease is almost nonexistent amongst some Eskimos.

The Oxford pioneer Hugh Sinclair who 'discovered' omega-3 oils found that taking 3 or 4 tablespoons of omega-3 oil daily increased bleeding time from small cuts on his arm from 30 seconds to 90 minutes, a graphic demonstration of the blood thinning effect of omega-3 oil.

DHA and EPA help modulate electrical activity in heart and brain cells and thus reduce risk of arrhythmia. Their important role in brain function has given rise to speculation that dietary supplementation with omega-3 fish oil might increase the intelligence of children. Indeed, use of omega-3 fish oils to treat depression has found that it increases brain size and it has been found that mothers who eat oily fish during pregnancy have children who are quicker at developing language skills.

[5] L-arginine

L-arginine helps promote production of nitric oxide (NO) in the endothelium (Cooke & Zimmer, 2002). In 1998 three Americans received a Nobel Prize for discovering that NO could act as a signal to many cells in the body and that NO was the 'endothelium-derived relaxing factor' (EDRF), a potent vasodilator that helps prevent hardening of the arteries by:
(a) Preventing blood platelet formation.
(b) Preventing white blood cells from sticking to blood vessel walls.
(c) Reducing production of free radicals which age blood vessels.
(d) Suppressing abnormal growth of vascular muscle cells which can thicken blood vessels.

Fish, nonfat milk products and nuts are rich in L-arginine.

A Harvard University study of 86,000 nurses found that those who ate more than five ounces of nuts per week lowered heart disease risk by 35% and a Californian study of over 31,000 people found that eating nuts five times a week halved risk of heart attack. Nuts are rich in L-arginine and also antioxidants including vitamin E and selenium, fibre, and monounsaturated oils similar to olive oil (Carper, 2000).

4. DIET DO'S AND DON'TS

[6] Garlic

Garlic has mild antiplatelet activity because it increases the activity of nitric oxide synthase. It also improves transport across cell membranes, reduces blood cholesterol levels, and helps clear the arteries,[2] research published online in 2010 in the journal *Maturitas* finding that taking four garlic extract capsules daily reduced blood pressure.

Garlic improves immune response and has mild antibacterial and antifungal properties. One study of 42,000 women found that those who consumed garlic in their diet were 30% less likely to develop colon cancer (Cooke & Zimmer, 2002). Another study found that garlic and grape seed supplements reduced risk of blood cancers.

Several herbs and some types of mushrooms are also thought to help prevent cancer (Varona, 2001).

[7] Soy

Soy products are rich in phytoestrogens and have been found to reduce cholesterol levels (Cooper, 1996) and one reason that the Japanese have half the cardiovascular disease of Americans may be their high consumption of soy (Cooke and Zimmer, 2002).

Soy also helps protect against cancer (Cooper, 1996) and men who eat plenty of soy are 72% less likely to develop lung cancer (*Journal of the American Medical Association* 294, 1493-1504, 2005).

Soy has also been found to be beneficial to post-menopausal women in a number of ways, including reduction of osteoporosis.

Lecithin, which is usually obtained from soy bean oil, is a phospholipid used to emulsify fats and, as discussed in Chapter 13, it has been found to reduce symptoms of heart and other diseases.

[8] Tea and cocoa

Tea is rich in antioxidants, especially a phytochemical called EGCG, green tea more so. Black tea protects against heart disease and green tea inhibits cancer growth and offers some protection against breast, ovarian and prostate cancer, reducing risk of the latter by two-thirds.

Tea has only half as much caffeine as coffee and a few cups daily should cause no problems except to those with high caffeine intolerance.

---

[2] In the first century AD Dioscorides proposed that garlic may help "clear the arteries" (Cooke & Zimmer, 2002). Feeding garlic to rabbits with 80% arterial blockage was found to reduce blockage (Carper, 2000).

Cocoa has very little caffeine and is three times richer in antioxidant flavonoids than green tea. Even as little as 6.3 gm of dark chocolate containing 30 mg of polyphenols has been found to reduce blood pressure in people with hypertension (Taubert D et al., *JAMA* 298 (2007) 49-60), but larger amounts should be avoided to keep fat intake low.

Caffeine stimulates the cerebral cortex and is a diuretic and thus lowers BP. The xanthines, theophylline in tea and theobromine in cocoa, have similar but less powerful effects.

[9] Plenty of fluids

Most authors recommend about eight 8-ounce glasses or 2 litres of water a day. Cooper (1996) cites a recommendation in *Tennis* magazine that you should have 9 (8 ounce) glasses of water a day if you weigh 115 pounds and do one hour of light exercise a day, but 9.5 glasses if you do moderate exercise and 10 glasses if you do strenuous exercise.

If you weigh 150 pounds 9 glasses a day are recommended for light exercise, 10 for moderate exercise, and 11.5 for strenuous exercise. If you weigh 200 pounds 9.5 glasses a day are recommended for light exercise, 11 for moderate exercise, and 13.25 for strenuous exercise.

Slightly higher levels of intake, however, will tend to thin the blood a little and thereby reduce blood cholesterol concentrations and thence vascular clogging.

Having plenty of fluids can also help flush out excess sodium at the risk, however, of also flushing out essential nutrients.

[10] Healthy snacks

It is best to eat about 8 times a day by having healthy snacks as well as three main meals. An example of this might be a study published in the *American Journal of Clinical Nutrition* which found that women who skipped breakfast had higher LDL levels and tended to eat more afterwards.

[11] Supplements

Regular vitamin C, E, Selenium and multivitamin supplements are strongly recommended for prevention and minimization of cancer and vascular disease.

Half an aspirin a day is also strongly recommended, at least for those older, as it has been well established that this reduces risk of heart attack, stroke and cancer.

Aspirin reduces inflammation and thence the risk of rupture of a plaque and release of blood clots. Thus for those with atherosclerosis-related concerns and raised levels of C-reactive protein, an indicator of inflammation in the body, low dosage of aspirin should be considered.

In contrast, a meta-analysis published in the British Medical Journal in 2011 found that 5 of the widely available non-steroidal anti-inflammatory drugs (NSAIDs) were associated with 2-4 times the risk of heart attack.

Things to minimize or avoid in your diet

[1] Fat

Some foods derived from animals are high in both fats and cholesterol, particularly red meat and cheese, and saturated fat intake also contributes significantly to blood cholesterol levels.

Saturated fat significantly increases the risk of heart disease and cancer. Therefore, the example diet of Chapter 26 has as little fat as possible, except for a quite large amount from peanuts which involve mostly healthy fats and are rich in L-arginine which, as noted earlier, promotes vascular health.

The journal *Nature* recently reported two US studies which showed that high-fat diets slowed learning and impaired memory in lab rats and mice. Conversely, rats given a drug that reduces triglyceride levels showed improved performance on memory tasks.

Approximately 5% of calories should be fat to provide enough fat for the body, for example to maintain cell membranes and endothelium linings, and to fuel basic brain and other functions.

Kurzweil (1993), however, showed that limiting fat calories to 10% reduced cholesterol levels very effectively and minimized risk of heart disease and cancer.

[2] Cholesterol

Daily cholesterol intake should be kept be below 300 mg, easily achieved if red meat and dairy foods are minimized. If you have a cholesterol problem or a personal or family history of heart disease you should limit cholesterol intake to 200 mg daily (Cooper, 1996).

Oxycholesterol found in fried and processed food, and especially in fast food, is a particularly damaging form of dietary cholesterol which should be avoided as far as possible.

[3] Sugar

Australian research published in the American Journal of Medicine in 2010 found that energy drinks increase blood platelet aggregation, leading to damage to blood vessel walls and greater risk of heart attack.

A 12-year Swedish study of 42,000 men found that drinking two fizzy soft drinks daily increased a man's risk of heart failure by 23 per cent.

A study of obese children aged 9 to 18 found that reducing sugar consumption, even without reducing overall calorie intake, lowered blood pressure and blood cholesterol in as little as nine days.

The WHO recommends that only 10% of calories come directly from sugars. Confectionery, soft drinks, biscuits, cakes and sweet desserts all contain a lot of sugar and thus have a high glycemic index (GI), a measure of how rapidly blood sugar levels rise after eating a food.

Glucose has GI = 100, honey has GI = 87 and white bread and candy bars have a GI of around 70. On the other hand, oatmeal has GI = 49 and oranges have GI = 42. Cherries, plums, grapefruit and peanuts have GI less than 30 (Sears, 1995) whilst soybeans have a GI of only 15 and contain immunity boosting phytoestrogens that keep blood vessels flexible and reduce the risk of hormone-related cancers (Somer, 2001).

[4] Sodium

Too much increases BP and a Canadian study found that for older people 4 days of high-salt diet halved arterial dilation (Carper, 2000). Thus the NHMRC and USFDA recommend a 2300 mg/day limit and the American Heart Association a 1500 mg/day limit.

Studies have shown that halving sodium intake reduces CVD and stroke by about 20-25%, but note that for some normotensive people low sodium intake increases CVD risk, whilst sweating from exercise and heat increases salt requirements considerably.

More potassium and less salt improves blood and lymph flow, helping remove waste deposits in the body, and one study found that a daily serving of potassium-rich food halved risk of stroke. Greater fluid intake also assists in waste removal, including excess salt (alkalizeforhealth.net).

[5] Food additives

Processed foods contain a wide variety of additives such as MSG for colour, flavour and preservation.. As discussed in Chapter 4, many of these involve health risks and some are carcinogenic (Eady, 2006).

4. DIET DO'S AND DON'TS

[6] Caffeine

Though alkaloid itself, caffeine increases acidity in the body, in turn promoting oxidation and production of free radicals. One study found that high coffee consumption increased risk of pancreatic cancer but, surprisingly, that people drinking only one or two cups of coffee a day had lower risk of pancreatic cancer (Kroger, 2005), a result comparable to the 'French paradox' of a little red wine reducing risk of heart disease.

Caffeine, however, is a stimulant which increases BP and pulse rate, undesirable in people with heart problems and therefore it should be limited.

Tea has much less caffeine than coffee and another alternative is cocoa which is rich in antioxidant flavonoids and procyanidins and has antioxidant properties up to twice as great as red wine and three times as great as green tea.

Flavonoids also reduce LDL levels and help prevent platelet build up in the blood. They also increase the flexibility of blood vessels and reduce the body's inflammatory responses which can trigger atherosclerosis.

[7] Alcohol

Most books on diet and heart disease note the many studies that indicate that a standard drink a day for women and one or two for men statistically reduces the probability of death from cardiovascular causes by from 20% to 40% or more.

Some of the reasons for this are thought to be:

(a) A blood-thinning property of alcohol.

(b) Its ability to increase HDL (Cooke and Zimmer, 2002). In fact, alcohol does not increase the important HDL2b responsible for reverse cholesterol transport (Superko, 2004).

(c) A possible anti-inflammatory effect, moderate drinkers having lower levels of C-reactive protein (CRP) in their blood, whereas levels of CRP are high in those at risk of heart disease. CRP is part of the body's response to inflammation and inflammation plays a major role in hardening of the arteries (Cooke and Zimmer, 2002).

Red wine is particularly recommended because it has potent antioxidants, particularly procyanidins (Corder, 2007), but also resveratrol and quercetin (Cooke and Zimmer, 2002).

Note that more than the very modest one or two daily drinks does more harm than good and results in increased incidence of heart disease and cancer. One reason for this is that significant quantities of alcohol raise triglyceride levels considerably and in turn risk of atherosclerosis.

A final warning. Pregnant women should have little or no alcohol rather than risk foetal brain damage as very small amounts of alcohol can have significant effect when body mass is very small. The same applies to smoking.

There are plenty of substitutes for alcohol such as fruit juice, ginger beer, sarsaparilla, and mixtures such as lemon, lime, bitters and soda.

[8] Too much acidity

Otto Warburg was awarded the Nobel Prize in 1931 for showing that the primary cause of cancer is lack of oxygen and thence greater fermentation of glucose within cells. In 1966 he found that a 35% decrease in oxygen caused embryonic cells to develop malignant characteristics. Current research confirms that excessive acidity reduces cellular oxygen levels (Varona, 2001).

Thus to minimize cancer risk diet plans should aim to avoid too much acidity increasing sugar, alcohol or caffeine and try to balance intake of mildly alkaline vegetables with intake of mildly acidic grains and breads.

It is important to remember that stress also increases acid levels, often resulting in stomach ulcers.

[9] Junk food

Fast food does provide many things needed in our diet but usually has "far too much fat" and too much salt and is lacking in fibre and many vitamins (Stanton, 1984).

A study published in the *American Journal of Clinical Nutrition* in 2005 revealed another down side.

This found that a breakfast of an Egg McMuffin and hash browns flooded the bloodstream with inflammatory components that make aneurysms more likely for 3 or 4 hours. A breakfast with the same number of calories but mostly of fruit and fibre, on the other hand, did not have the same inflammatory effect.

More alarmingly, a six-year study of 17,000 people found that people who ate lots of fried food and sugary drinks have a 56 per cent higher risk of heart disease.

4. Diet Do's and Don'ts

[10] 'Gassy' eating habits
One possible result of eating lots of vegetables, especially beans, is 'gas' or flatulence. Varona (2001) makes a number of suggestions as to how this problem might be reduced:

(a) Don't eat too much and chew your food thoroughly.

(b) Limit intake of beans and add salt to improve their digestion.

(c) Have a break before eating dessert so that simple sugars do not end up fermenting slower-digesting grains. Some people might even find eating proteins and carbohydrates separately helps too.

(d) Avoid stress and limit fluid intake after meals.

Table 4.2. Do's and don'ts of some common foods.

	Do	Don't
Fat	Skim milk	Butter, cheese and margarine
	Fish & fish oils	Animal fat
	Baked beans	Chocolate (a little dark chocolate is OK)
	Cereals & grains	Potato crisps & like snacks
	Fresh fruit	Fried food
	Fresh vegetables	Eggs
Salt	Salt reduced bread	Use salt in cooking
	Fresh fruit	Canned vegetables
	Potatoes & rice	Condiments & salad dressings
	Pasta	Frozen/packaged meals
	Nuts (unsalted)	Potato crisps & like snacks
	Tea & coffee	Canned vegetable juice
Sugar	Dry biscuits, bread	Confectionery, sugar, soft drinks
	Grains & cereals	Jam & syrup
	Vegetables	Sweet biscuits & cake
Fibre	Wholemeal bread	White bread
	Brown rice	White rice

Table 4.2 uses some common foods as examples of what foods to have, and what foods not to have, in relation to fat, sodium, sugar, and fibre.

4. Diet Do's and Don'ts

Vitamins

Table 4.3 lists some foods rich in some of the more important vitamins and minerals. The third column suggests dietary supplementation for most nutrients, especially more elusive vitamins like B12 and E, and to cover the B-complex range and incorporate important minerals like selenium.

Table 4.3. Food sources of the most important vitamins.

Vitamin/mineral	Good food sources	Suggestion
A	Liver, orange fruit & veg. green leafy vegetables	Get via carotenoids in fruit & vegetables
B1	Wholegrain cereals and meats, esp. pork	Diet + multivitamin or B-complex tablets
B2	Milk, meats, green leafy vegetables	"
B3 (niacin)	Meats & eggs, milk	"
B6	All foods	"
B12	Offal the richest source	"
C	Citrus fruits	Fruit + tablets
D	Only in fortified food	From sun
E	Vegetable oils, corn, soybean	Vegetables + tablets/capsules
Folic Acid	Green leafy vegetables, fruits, liver & kidney	Diet + tablets
Calcium	Milk, including skim milk	Skim milk + tablets
Potassium	Fruits & vegetables	Fruits & vegetables
Magnesium	Cereals, cocoa	Tablets
Iodine	Iodized salt	Multivitamin & mineral tablets
Iron	Red meats, esp. liver	Tablets or MV tablets
Selenium	Sea foods, meat	Tablets or MV tablets
Zinc	Seafood, especially oysters	Tablets or MV tablets

4. Diet Do's and Don'ts

For those concerned with iron-deficiency anaemia iron supplements are beneficial (for pernicious anaemia B12 is needed) whilst zinc supplementation may be helpful with benign prostate enlargement symptoms.

Note in passing that the body excretes excess vitamin B2, making urine yellow, which the author takes as a good sign, and that most vitamins tend to boost the immune system (Bock & Sabin, 1997).

As 'general insurance', the occasional multivitamin tablet is also worthwhile and recommended by most doctors.

More on meat

One US study concluded that eating meat three times a week doubled the risk of CVD.

According to Michael Mosley, who recently tested the effect of increased meat consumption on his health, modest consumption of meat daily (he tried 85 gm of various meats such as pork daily for a few weeks) is OK and saturated fat is not quite as great a villain as once thought.

Myself, just looking at a large 1 kilo lump of partly yellowed and solidified saturated fat is enough to convince me that it will certainly tend to clog my arteries, but perhaps not as badly as once thought as much of it might not be absorbed by the body and just go 'straight through' almost and be excreted.

Mosley found that after 4 weeks of his modest meat diet his cholesterol levels remained OK, and his blood pressure likewise.

The catch with red meat, it is now thought, is it's L-carnitine which reacts with bacteria who 'eat' it in the stomach, then excretes a more deleterious chemical to be absorbed in the intestines, and this chemical encourages and/or facilitates the formation of plaque, however.

Indeed, animal tests do confirm that increased consumption of L-carnitine does result in greater incidence of CVD. Moreover, a 30-year Harvard study of 120,000 people did show that increased consumption of red meat did result in higher incidence of CVD and cancer, 35 g/day increasing risk of death by 13%, whilst the same amount of processed meat (i.e., bacon, ham and sausages) per day increased risk by 20%.

Processed meat is the greater villain because it contains extra salt and sodium nitrite as a result of processing, the nitrite being converted by the body to nitrosamines, polyaromatic hydrocarbons (PAHs) comparable to those that result from tobacco smoking, and these give greater risk of cancer.

So the bottom line, according to Mosley, is that a little red meat (say once a week), is OK, but otherwise lighter meats like chicken are preferred, while processed meats should be avoided as far as possible (Mosley, 2015).

Conclusion

Eliminate fat and thence most cheese, meat, chocolate and snack foods. Substitute fat free or fat reduced products such as skim milk.

Increase fibre, for example high fibre cereals or baked beans, to reduce absorption of fats in food.

Increase fruit and vegetables to obtain nutrition, fibre and antioxidants.

Eat fish rich in omega-3 oils to combat heart disease.

Include garlic to help reduce blood cholesterol.

Include foods rich in phytosterols such as kidney beans in your meals as these help reduce cholesterol absorption.

Include food rich in antioxidants such as carrots and other highly coloured fruit and vegetables which are rich in carotenoids.

Reduce sugar in the diet to help reduce triglyceride levels.

Reduce salt in the diet to avoid vascular inflammation.

Reduce total calorie intake to lose body fat and thence weight.

Limit yourself to an evening 'tipple' of just a couple of drinks. This is said to increase HDL, but not HDL2b responsible for reverse cholesterol transport. Red wine has useful antioxidants, particularly the procyanidins (Corder, 2007), and the reason why two or three drinks, but not more, is beneficial is discussed in Chapter 10.

Drink tea, rich in antioxidants (especially green tea). A study of women in the 70s and 80s found that those who drank two cups of tea daily were 40 per cent less likely to die during the five years of the study.

If you smoke give it up as a high priority.

This, however, is only the start of the story. We haven't talked about cholesterol much yet, for example. Nor have we talked about exercise.

These and other topics are dealt with in following chapters, including good advice on how to give up smoking in Chapter 8.

4. Diet Do's and Don'ts

Chapter 5

HARMFUL FOOD ADDITIVES

Have you ever wondered why we have increasing rates of childhood illness despite increasing amounts of money we put into our health system? Do you wonder why rates of cancer, ADHD, depression, suicide, and even cardiovascular disease continue to rise in children? The reason is clear. We do not have a system that creates health. We have a pharmaceutical based health system that treats the symptoms and not the disease.
Julie Eady, *Additive Alert*, 2nd edn, (2006)

MSG

There are a host of food additives in use today, the list growing ever longer year by year, often without new additives having had sufficient research to test them for adverse effects.

MSG, i.e., monosodium glutamate (621), is an additive about which negative publicity over the last decade or two has led to some public awareness that intake of this substance should be limited.

MSG is the sodium salt of glutamic acid, a tasteless white powder with no nutritional value that is used as a flavour enhancer. It has been found to cause asthma, hyperactivity, depression, mood changes, sleeplessness, nausea, migraine, and has been linked to infertility, congenital abnormalities, convulsions, and abdominal discomfort.

Glutamate is a neurotransmitter belonging to the *excitotoxins* group of amino acids which includes cysteine and aspartate. Excessive amounts of these cause overstimulation and kill brain cells.

In 1969 MSG was prohibited from use in baby foods in the US after research found that it caused detrimental effects on the brains and nervous systems of young animals, and that pregnant monkeys and rats fed MSG gave birth to brain-damaged infants.

More recently MSG in amounts little more than those in human foods was found to increase appetite in rats by 40%, perhaps accounting in part for the obesity epidemic that faces us now.

Often other glutamates than 621, such as 620, 622, 623, 624, 625, 627, 631 and 635 are used, but these have the same adverse effects as MSG, and in same cases additional negative effects.

Worse still, *Hydrolysed Vegetable Protein*, a concentrated form of natural MSG is often used, and this contains known carcinogens. Many other food additives such as 'plant protein extract' and 'yeast extract' also contain MSG, while even 'spices' may do so (Eady, 2006).

Artificial sweeteners

Aspartame (951), also an excitotoxin, is an artificial sweetener the safety of which was hotly debated for 20 years before it was approved in the US, despite data linking it to brain tumour development in rats.

"Aspartame is considered by some to be the most dangerous substance on the market that is added to foods. It accounts for 75% of the adverse reactions reported to the USFDA" (Eady, 2006).

Reported adverse effects range from migraines to tachycardia and memory loss. Most important, like MSG it can damage brain cells, of which damage foetuses and infants are at most risk.

An Italian study completed in 2005 found that dosages similar to the intake limit set for humans caused lymphomas and leukemia in female animals (Eady, 2006).

Other common sweeteners also have deleterious effects, for example:

(a) Acesulphame Potassium (950) and saccharin (954) cause cancer in animals and for humans the latter is classified as a weak carcinogen.

(b) Tests have found sucralose (955) to cause kidney and liver damage and it has been linked to neurological and immunological disorders.

Nitrates and nitrites

Salt-like sodium nitrate and sodium nitrite are added to processed meats as a preservative to enhance colour and flavour.

Nitrites affect oxygenation of the blood and are not allowed in foods intended for infants or young children. This effect can be counteracted by antioxidants such as vitamins C and E.

Nitrates and nitrites react with amines in meats to form *nitrosamines* which are "hazardous poisons and definite animal carcinogens" and "widely considered to be toxic and carcinogens in humans" (Eady, 2006).

A survey of 12 common consumer products said of beef frankfurters: *Children eating up to about a dozen each month are at an approximately four-fold increased risk of brain cancer and seven-fold increased risk of leukemia."* (Eady, 2006).

Artificial colours

The best known negative effect of these is hyperactivity, especially in young children, this mainly applying to Coal Tar and AZO dyes including 102, 104, 110, 122, 123, 124, 132, 133, 142 and 155 (Eady, 2006).

In the last 20 years more than a dozen food dyes have been pulled from the market because of lab findings that they were carcinogenic.

Several others with links to cancer, including Amaranth (123), Food Green (142), Brilliant Black (151), Carbon Black (153) and Brown HR (155) are banned in other countries but still allowed in Australia.

Annatto (160b), often found in cheese and margarine, is associated with behavioural and learning difficulties in children.

Tartrazine (102), found in many foods including juices, causes mood, gastric, and sleep problems. Tartrazine is one of several dyes, along with caramel (150), used to make so-called chocolate coated biscuits without cocoa (Eady, 2006).

Preservatives

Preservatives are found in most foods, including such staples as bread, fruit juice, margarine, and even supposedly fresh meats and fish.

Some preservatives involve health risks, examples being:

(a) Sulphites (220-228).

These release sulphur dioxide, causing asthmatics difficulty and "220 is a suspected mutagen and possible teratogen" (Eady, 2006).

(b) Proprionates (280-283).

These cause gastric, migraine, mood, sleep, behaviour and learning problems and calcium proprionate (282) is banned in the UK because it causes skin rashes in bakers.

(c) Benzoates (210-213).

These are deemed dangerous for asthmatics and cause hyperactivity, skin and gastric problems. Sodium benzoate is linked with kidney, liver and neural toxicity, also being a suspected teratogen.

In 2006 US and UK authorities found high levels of benzene residue in popular brands of soft drink, perhaps a result of heat and/or light stimulated reaction of sodium or potassium benzoate with vitamin C. Benzene and acridine (used in making dyes and drugs) are both DNA mutants and thus carcinogenic (Galton, 2001).

Dried and fresh fruit

Dried fruit usually has sulphur dioxide (202) as a preservative and this may pose concerns for asthmatics.

Fresh fruit and nuts are often coated with the neurotoxin propylene glycol (1520) to retain moisture but this is toxic and linked to kidney and liver damage (Eady, 2006).

Antioxidants

These are used widely, especially in products that contain oils or fats, and thus may have cumulative effects. Most antioxidants are safe but 310, 311, 312, 319, 320, and 321 are suspected of being a danger to asthmatics and should be avoided,

Propyl, octyl and dodecyl-gallate (310-312) irritate asthmatics and are suspected carcinogens.

Tert-butylhydroquinone (319) or TBHQ is a suspected carcinogen and teratogen and can also cause nausea, vomiting, delirium and collapse, 5 grams of TBHQ being fatal to an adult.

Butylated hydroxyanisole (320) or BHA has cumulative effects and is a known animal carcinogen that also disrupts hormone balance. BHA is found in sweet and savoury biscuits, margarine, peanut butter, mayonnaise, ice-cream cones and frozen foods, despite being prohibited for foods intended for infants or young children.

Butylated hydroxytoluene or BHT (321) is a "proven teratogen and carcinogen" in animals and suspected of being likewise in humans (Eady, 2006).

5. Harmful Food Additives

Conclusion

Clearly modern use of food additives had got out of hand, there being far too many suspect ones for comfort, whilst several, at least, are downright dangerous, especially over the long term when they have cumulative effects.

Pregnant women and very young children should avoid MSG whilst we should all avoid additives that have been proven carcinogenic in animal or human trials.

Asthmatics need to take extra care as many food additives appear at least a slight risk of causing irritation, if not more serious symptoms.

Many processed food such as potato chips, cookies, doughnuts and fried fast foods are loaded with unnatural and unhealthy saturated fats, whereas natural fats such as those found in olives, nuts and fish are healthy, particularly the omega-3 fatty acids which are good for our hearts and our brains.

Countless other processed foods, of course, are high in salt and (refined) sugar.

Another concern with the processing of foods is the great loss of nutrients, for example:

➢ 48.9% of B6 is lost in processing seafood.
➢ 77% of B6 is lost in processing vegetables.
➢ Up to 78% of pantothenic acid is lost in food processing.
➢ 86.5% of vitamin E and 50% of molybdenum is lost in wheat refining.
➢ 81.7% of manganese, 70.6% of cobalt, and 40% of zinc are lost in canned spinach.
➢ 50% of choline is lost in refining brown rice (Somer, 2001).

Little wonder then, that vitamin deficiencies are often to blame for some of our many ailments.

The solution to the dangers of processed foods involves a number of elements, including:

(1) Eat healthy foods such as whole grains, fruit, vegetables, and fish.

(2) Avoid foods high in fat, especially saturated and trans fats.[1]

(3) Avoid butter and margarine as much as possible, for example by making a jam sandwich with just jam. It should taste better.

---

[1] On 15/6/2018 Australian news media reported that health authorities were considering banning the use of trans fats in manufactured food.

(4) Consume plenty of fibre to help carry away excess dietary fat.

(5) Avoid food high in salt and sugar.

(6) Take at least a few vitamin supplements regularly.

(7) Drink plenty of fluids including water, weak tea, and coffee (the latter in moderation) to help rinse out excesses of things like salt.

As for food additives, these are often not shown or are represented misleadingly on product labels. Ingredients lists are usually in such fine print that most older people will need not only glasses, but perhaps a magnifying glass as well to decipher them, an exercise really only practical at home but better late than never, of course.

Chapter 6

LOSING WEIGHT

> *Women who are overweight when they are diagnosed*
> *with breast cancer are twice as likely to die*
> *of the disease as women who are of normal weight.*
> Study published in *Journal of Clinical Oncology* (2004).

Calorie counting

In Chapter 4 there is a table (Table 4.1) of calorie values for a small selection of foods. The key to any weight loss and control program is a calorie counter booklet such as Alan Borushek's pocket-sized but invaluable *Calorie Counter* (2014).

With the aid of this little book you can quickly find out the calorie content of any food and drink that you have. Then you should write down what you ate and total your calories for each day in your diary.

This can be compared to the number of calories appropriate for your ideal weight. Your ideal weight can be determined from the formulas

Men:

45 kg for 150 cm in height + 1.05 kg per cm taller   (6.1)

or   105 lb for first 5 ft in height + 6 lb per inch taller

Women:

43 kg for 150 cm in height + 0.9 kg per cm taller   (6.2)

or   100 lb for first 5 ft in height + 5 lb per inch taller

For example, a man of 183 cm in height should be 80 kg. This is at the top of the 5 - 8 kg range for a man with a 'medium' frame. For a small frame subtract about 5 kg, for a large frame add about 6 kg.

A woman 173 cm in height should be 64 kg. This is around the lower end of the 5 - 7 kg range for a woman with a 'medium' frame. For a small frame subtract about 4 kg and for a large frame add about 5 kg.

6. Losing Weight

If you prefer Imperial units then a man 6 feet in height should be 177 pounds and a woman 5 feet 8 inches in height should be 140 pounds.

These formulae are approximate only and if they are too much for you refer to the charts in such books as Borushek's calorie counter (2014).

Now you must calculate the calorie intake appropriate for your ideal weight. You can do this using for following formula

Women: 1550 calories for 45 kg in weight + 20 cals/kg extra

or   6500 kJ for 45 kg in weight + 84 kJ/kg extra

For men add 500 calories.

This is for people in the age range 35 - 55. If you are older than this subtract about 300 calories and if you are younger than this (but more than 18) add about 300 calories.

For example, a woman of 45 who weighs 60 kg (for whom correct height according to Eqn 7.2 is 169 cm) requires

1550 + 15 X 20 = 1850 calories

A man of 45 who weighs 75 kg (for whom correct height according to Eqn 6.1 is 179 cm) requires

1550 + 500 + 30 X 20 = 2050 + 600 = 2650 calories

Note in passing a piece of trivia. We are supposed to have about six pints of blood. 2000 calories is enough to boil that amount of water about five times.

As the adjustments for age range might suggest, allowance should also be made for your level of activity. If you are bedridden subtract from 500 to 900 calories depending upon your weight and a similar adjustment might be made for a crash diet (which I do not recommend at all).

If you are moderately active physically by way of your daily activities, for example in the skilled trades, add 250 to 450 calories depending upon your weight. If you are highly active, for example a professional sports person, add from 500 to 900 calories depending upon your weight.

Well now, by way of the foregoing formulas, or from tables in countless books and magazines, you should be able to estimate your ideal weight and thence the appropriate calorie intake.

Body mass index

In losing weight the objective should be to get a couple of kilograms below the 'ideal weight' recommended by Eqns 6.1 or 6.2, also aiming to make sure that your body mass index, that is

$$BMI = (weight\ in\ kg)/(height\ in\ metres)^2$$

is somewhere around 20.

It may take months or even years to get BMI down to this conservative target figure but the objective is to eliminate excess body fat and a simple skinfold test[1] should be the final guide as to whether you have reached this goal.

The aim here is to help ensure, that along with appropriate diet and plenty of exercise, your body will burn up much of the cholesterol deposits that began to clog your blood vessels early in life.

The potential benefits are enormous:

[1] When you finally reach your 'fighting weight' you will, of course, be fighting fit, particularly as along the way you have become accustomed to a healthy diet and plenty of exercise.

[2] You will have reduced your statistical risk of vascular disease and cancer by around 50%.

[3] If you have already had symptoms of vascular disease, you should have been able to reduce these, if you started soon enough perhaps avoiding the need for major heart surgery later in life.

[4] A 1997 World Cancer Research Fund report concluded that 30 to 40% of cancers could be avoided with appropriate diet, regular exercise and not being overweight (Corder, 2007).

[5] If you are unlucky enough to be diagnosed with cancer then making your diet a little stricter along the lines of the Moerman Therapy and taking larger doses of vitamins A, C, E and selenium (see Table 18.1) might help you beat the disease, along with specialist treatment, of course.

---

[1] The skinfold test site for men is the waistline, for women either the buttocks or upper arms (Sudy, 1991). Special calipers can be used for accurate skinfold measurements (Marchese & Hill, 2005).

6. Losing Weight

A case study

I started to calculate calories seriously during my final (and successful) quit smoking effort, concerned about not putting on too much weight, as people usually are when quitting because they are apt, quite rightly, to eat more, in part as a substitute for smoking.

Then I made sure that I was providing myself with, if anything, extra calories to make sure there were no additional cravings other than for cigarettes occasionally (in any event there were remarkably few of these, even from the outset). Thus, for example, I was happy to have a few extra drinks in the evening, indeed encouraging myself to have that next drink rather than even pause to think of a cigarette, thus breaking the quite common and strong association between smoking and alcohol, perhaps because they are somewhat self-canceling as nicotine is a stimulant and alcohol a tranquilizer.

Thanks to a little calorie counting and plenty of exercise, however, I did not gain weight.

Then, when I was finally sure that I had indeed finally rid myself of the horrible smoking habit, I decided to lose weight as I was about 8 pounds above correct weight, being 6'2" tall, just above 13 stone, and consuming about 2800 calories a day to maintain that weight.

To lose weight I simply had to set a lower daily calorie target!

I noted that you have to burn about 3500 calories in energy in order to lose about a pound (0.45 kg) in weight. I decided that I'd like to lose something like a pound a week if possible and that translated to reducing mys calorie intake by about 500 calories daily, giving me a target of 2300 calories daily.

Table 6.1 is an example of the simple bachelor diet I had in order to lose weight, in conjunction with up to a couple of hours walking daily.

I did indeed find that I lost up to a pound a week, depending upon how much walking I did, so that after a few weeks I had reached my target weight. Then I maintained my weight-loss routine for a few more months until I was about ten pounds below target.

In the end I lost about 21 pounds (10 kilos roughly) and was 11 stone 5 pounds or 72 kilos, at the bottom of the range for my height and around the weight I had been in my early twenties. After decades of physical lethargy there was barely any to muscle to lose so it had been even more important to minimize excess fat.

64

Table 6.1. A simple weight-loss diet.

Meal	Food	Calories
Breakfast	wheat flakes + milk	175
	fruit juice	75
Lunch	meat pie	400
	sardines on toast	400
Dinner	tuna & rice	400
	apple pie	150
Evening	3 glasses wine or fruit juice	250
	biscuits & tea	250
	hot chocolate & cake	150
Sundry	other tea & coffee	50
	+ minimum sugar	
TOTAL		2300

Over the next decade my weight stayed about the same until around the time I began work on my first health book (Mohr, 2012b). Then I began working on the diet and exercise programs outlined in this book and lost a few more pounds so that I had hardly any excess fat left and was then, if anything, at least a couple of pounds underweight.

Fasting

Some religious people practice fasting for one day each week, often their 'Sabbath' day. Most people who do practice fasting for religious or other reasons, however, also make sure of feeding themselves up the day before and catching up on any calorie shortfall the following day as well. Indeed, many might well have a binge the day after fasting.

For that reason, to be successful weight-loss diets must involve a fairly constant daily dose of calories.

One might be moved to wonder whether fasting, however, might not be an effective way of reducing blood cholesterol levels and perhaps cholesterol plaques in our arteries. The author is inclined to think, on the other hand, that increased levels of exercise and the various diet and dietary supplements measures discussed in later chapters might be the better course to take.

Conclusion

To lose weight work out the number of calories appropriate for your sex, height and build. Then subtract enough from that number to lose, for example, a kilo in two or three weeks.

If you are overweight you have probably not being doing enough exercise so you need to do a substantial amount of exercise to help shed weight and this is discussed in the next chapter.

It might also help if you substitute healthy grains and fruit and vegetables for foods high in fat or sugar. The importance of doing this to reduce the vascular damage of cholesterol and homocysteine is discussed in later chapters.

Finally, there are many benefits from losing weight, self-esteem being perhaps the least important. More important are such benefits as reduced risk of heart attack, stroke and cancer.

An example of this was provided by research on the health records of 2314 men between the ages of 50 and 70 (E. Ingelsson et al., *Heart* 2006). The results showed that those with *metabolic syndrome,* a combination of obesity, high blood pressure, high blood fat levels and diabetes, had twice as many heart attacks.

This finding is in part explained by the fact that *"carrying even a few extra pounds can significantly increase your total cholesterol, including your 'bad' cholesterol"* (Cooper, 1996) so that weight loss is crucial.

An example of the many other benefits of losing weight is reduction of problems with arthritis. According to a study published in the *Journal of Arthritis & Rheumatism* (vol. 52, pp 2026-33, 2005), every 500 g of weight lost took nearly 2 kg of load off the knees.

Perhaps the most dramatic example of the benefits of losing weight, it has been found that calorific restriction to the extent of 30% fewer calories in insects, mice, rabbits, dogs, cats, and monkeys, increases their life span by 30%. This increase may be in part owing to the SIR_2 gene, one of many which counteract the aging process that have been found in yeast cells, fruit flies, and worms.

Many further examples of studies which show the negative effects on health that come from being overweight are given in following chapters. On a more positive note, a great many studies which show the benefits of healthy diet and exercise are also discussed in following chapters, hopefully providing motivation for those who need to lose weight.

Chapter 7

EXERCISE

> *Research by Dr Lemole has demonstrated that*
> *the flow of lymph prevents and removes atherosclerosis.*
> *The flow of lymph is accelerated by exercise - -*
> www.alkalizeforhealth.net/Lymphsystem.htm
> Referring to a book by Lemole and Gerald (2000).

The need for exercise

I recall a time when older people were advised to do a 10 minute walk daily. This is pathetically inadequate and, indeed, a high proportion of older people hardly do that.

The result is that their muscles waste away and, in the end, they are unable to walk without aids, then ultimately bedridden.

In fact it is tragic to see the elderly literally waste away in this way when little more than token efforts at calisthenics, walking, on an exercise bike, and with small weights, would make a dramatic difference to their health, as many scientific studies have found.

An absolute minimum, therefore, should be about half an hour walking daily, or the equivalent. Some more intensive exercise should also be done, if possible without risk, as this may be more beneficial for heart and general health because it exercises other muscles and opens up tired arteries more.

The need for care

Those unused to exercise for some time should, of course, take care to gradually build up their efforts (Bingham & Hadfield, 2007). In addition, when doing particularly strenuous exercises such as those involving heavy weights (in relation to one's physical strength), great care must be taken to warm up one's body and, in particular, heart a little with some light exercise.

Studies on the health benefits of exercise

[1] Exercise increases arterial flexibility, decreases blood pressure, increases 'good' HDL levels, and decreases 'bad 'LDL levels. Exercise also increases levels of the antioxidant enzyme superoxide dismutase [SOD] (Cooke, 2002). Low levels of SOD are found in patients with heart failure whereas increasing SOD levels can reverse atherosclerosis (Nicholas J, Life Extension Magazine, Oct. 2008).

[2] The 12 month Heidelberg Regression Study found that combination of a 20% of calories from fat diet (< 50% of fat saturated), and 5-6 hours of 'training' exercise per week, could prevent progression of heart disease (Shuler et al., 1992). Retrospective statistical analysis of the data showed that 1000 calories of exercise a week allowed progression of the disease but that 1500 calories stabilized it, and 2000 - 2200 calories or more gave regression (Gielen et al., 2001; Superko, 2004).

Notably, the 2000 calories exercise level is that used in Kurzweil's 10% solution for preventing heart disease and cancer (Kurzweil, 1993) which, as shown in Table 16.2, greatly reduces blood cholesterol levels.

[3] A study of exercise benefits in heart disease by Gielen et al. (2001) found that:

(a) Exercise training reduces blood viscosity and just 4 weeks of exercise training reduces vasoconstriction.

(b) Exercise increases production of artery-relaxing nitric oxide (NO) and its half-life (probably quite rapidly), giving greater vasodilation in response to blood flow or the neurotransmitter acetylcholine.

(c) 16 weeks of exercise training of pigs improved microvasculature (minor heart blood vessels of 0.3 mm diameter or less), thus increasing total vascular bed cross-sectional area by 37%, reducing vascular resistance and increasing maximal flow reserve.[1]

(d) Animal studies showed that long-term intensive physical exercise improved coronary collateralization.

(e) Exercise training of pigs increased adenosine-mediated arteriolar permeability for serum albumin by 65%, indicating higher vascular permeability.

(f) Despite involving some risk, exercise training gives a nett benefit in reducing thrombogenic risk in coronary artery disease.

---

[1] c.f. coronary arteries of marathon runners are 2 to 3 times normal size and have much greater capacity to expand (Cooke & Zimmer, 2002).

7. Exercise

[4] Infections are the leading cause of death in people aged 65 and over, and a 2008 article in JAMA found that moderate exercise increases immunity by improving the function of neutrophils which initiate the immune response and combat foreign micro-organisms, and by increasing numbers and functioning of immune system cells such as the 'natural killer' (NK) cell (Tzar C, *The Weekend Australian* Jan 19-12 2008).

[5] A study published in 2008 in an American physiology journal found that exercise reduced inflammatory response in wounds and thus improved healing, an important finding in relation to inflammation-related diseases, including arthritis, type-2 diabetes, heart disease and Alzheimer's disease (Tzar C, *The Weekend Australian* Jan 19-12 2008).

[6] A survey of 284 members of a running club and a control group of 156 people, all being over 50 at the start of the study, found that after 19 years 34% of the non-runners had died, whereas the runners had fewer disabilities and only 15% had died (Chakravarty EF et al., *Arch Intern Med* 168 (2008) 1638-1646).

[7] A 5-year study of 3200 people over 65 published in the 2009 British Medical Journal found that those who walked slowest were 1.4 times more likely to die, and 2.9 times more likely to die of heart disease.

[8] The interstitial fluid or lymph provides oxygen and nutrients to the cells and carries carbon dioxide, acid wastes, dead cells, bacteria and viruses away. It has also been found that lymph flow can remove atheroma (Lemole & Gerald, 2000). A benefit of aerobic exercise is that lymph circulation is improved by both deep breathing and exercise.

[9] A 20-year study published in 2010 found that of 95,396 post-menopausal women, those who walked an hour daily had 15% lesser risk of breast cancer than those who only walked an hour a week.
A study of 3000 women diagnosed with breast cancer found walking 3-5 hours/week cut death rates by 50% (*J AMA* 2005: 293(20) 2479-86).

[10] Two studies of patients with bowel cancer found that those who were physically active reduced recurrence and mortality rates by 50-60% (*Clinical Oncology* 24 (2006) 3527; 3535).

[11] Men aged 65 or older who do at least three hours a week of vigorous exercise lowered their risk of high grade, advanced or fatal prostate cancer by almost 70 per cent according to a 2005 article in *Archives of Internal Medicine* (vol. 165, pp 1005-1010).

[12] Exercise has also been found to reduce the side effects of cancer treatment (*Support Cancer Care* 14 (2006) 732).

[13] A UCLA study of mice showed that a combination of exercise and L-arginine and vitamin C and E supplements increased nitric oxide (NO) levels, making them far less likely to suffer internal damage to their arteries (BBC news online, 28/4/2004).

[14] A 14-year study of 123,000 people published in the *American Journal of Epidemiology* in 2010 found that women who sat for 6 hours a day had 34% greater death risk than those who sat for 3 hours, the figure for men sitting 6 hours/day being 17% increase.

[15] One study found that women exercising vigourously enough to cause sweating or fast heartbeat for just 20 minutes two or three times a week were 20 percent less likely to suffer from heart problems, stoke and blood clots than inactive women. Those who did gentler exercise such as walking, cycling or gardening had the same reduction in risk (Herald Sun, Melbourne, 18/2/2015).

There have been many such findings and Superko (2004) concludes: "Exercising 7 days a week for an hour each session is my Prescription for everyone with existing coronary heart disease," citing the Heidelberg study as a "compelling" argument for this recommendation.

Heart rate

The idea is that you are supposed to get up to your maximum heart rate to achieve much by way of benefit. In fact, it is sufficient to get into your target range, perhaps building up from the lower end of the range to the higher end over a few weeks.

Then the objective of a good exercise program is that it should involve exercise sessions three or four times a week which involve getting your heart rate into its target range at least three times in each session.

Motivation for this, an 18-year study of 50,000 people published in *Journal of Epidemiology and Community Health* in 2010 found that, except for women over 70, those with higher resting heart rates were more likely to die of heart disease. For men over 70 risk increased by about 10% for each increment of 10 in resting heart rate while for women under 70 risk rose by 18%.

7. EXERCISE

Table 7.1 gives maximum and target heart rate ranges for various ages calculated from the simple formula: Maximum HR = 220 - Age
and target heart range is 65 - 85% of the maximum HR (Kurzweil, 1993).

Table 7.1. Maximum and target heart rates for various ages.

Age	Maximum HR	Target HR
20	200	130 - 170
25	195	127 - 166
30	190	124 - 162
35	185	120 - 157
40	180	117 - 153
45	175	114 - 149
50	170	111 - 145
55	165	107 - 140
60	160	104 - 136
65	155	101 - 132
70	150	98 - 128
75	145	94 - 123

A 5-year study of 9190 people published online in *European Heart Journal* found that those with HR > 84 had 55% greater risk of cardiovascular death and 79% greater risk of death from any cause.

Weights

We should all get about 30 minutes aerobic exercise such as walking or running per day. This need not be all in one go and it is just as beneficial to have, say, two 15 minute sessions.

We should also work against resistance to maintain or rebuild muscle, preferably using weights, a good example being strap-on ankle weights used by sitting in a chair and raising the weighted leg up straight numerous times, a good exercise to help keep older people walking OK.

Muscle is built by slowly stretching muscle fibers. This causes microscopic damage to some of the muscle fibres and as a result *satellite cells* are formed. These fuse with the damaged fibres to produce stronger and bigger muscles, and desirably you should have a break of a day or two between resistance workouts on the same muscles to allow them 'recovery and building time.'

7. Exercise

Weights are used to build muscle and, as 5 kilos of muscle will burn an extra 150 calories a day, this will help you lose body fat more quickly if you need to.

As a crude example, a short barbell session with moderate weights might be three sets of 10 - 30 repetitions of the following exercises:

[1] Above head lifts.

[2] Barbell curls (forearms moving from horizontal to vertical).

[3] Squats holding the barbell.

Such a routine should quickly get you into your target HR and keep it there, particularly if there is not much break between the three 'elements' of the routine.

Building up strength

A typical program for building up strength using weights might be:

Week 1: 3 sets of 15 reps per exercise. Rest 30 seconds between reps. Do the reps slowly without jerking the weights.

Week 2: 5 sets of 15 reps

Week 3: 7 sets of 15 reps

Week 4: 3 sets of 12 reps with increased weight.

Week 5: 5 sets of 12 reps

Week 6: 7 sets of 12 reps

Week 7: 3 sets of 8 reps with increased weight

Week 8: 5 sets of 8 reps

Week 9: 7 sets of 8 reps

Week 10: Repeat week 1, now with increased weight.

Many people might be satisfied with two weight increments. If so, they would stop at the week 9 routine and simply maintain that.

The numbers of reps mentioned here pertain to modest weights which can be purchased economically at discount stores for home use.

Note that the foregoing program is designed to increase strength. For endurance and heart health it is better to aim at larger numbers of reps and lower weights (Cooke and Zimmer, 2002).

For older people the weights might be minimal, for example the small plastic coated dumbbells that power walkers use.

Here, however, a note of caution. Researchers at the University of Florida found that carrying hand weights while walking can increase blood pressure (Prevention Magazine, 1991). That's good for weight loss and cardiovascular endurance but perhaps a risk for people with blood pressure problems.

Home gym apparatus with a bench and weights operated though pulleys is also quite affordable. With this equipment there is no problem is you drop the weights.

Needless to say, the same sort of 'build up' used in weight training can also be applied to walking and running routines where distance or speed can be increased.

This is a good point at which to remember the old adage about moderation in all things. Rowers competing at the highest levels for several years in which they are forced to work above their 'own rate' run the risk of an enlarged and permanently damaged heart.

The catalogue of permanent injuries that can be sustained in sport is too long to consider here, but the moral is that exercise for the sake of health should be moderate and carefully thought out and done.

Conclusion

The purposes and benefits of exercise include:

[1] To lose weight and replace fat with muscle.

[2] To reduce blood triglyceride and LDL levels, increase HDL levels, and thus reduce cholesterol deposits in your vascular system, including in the capillaries in your eyes and brain. Blood sugar levels are also reduced, reducing risk of diabetes.

[3] To strengthen heart muscle to reduce the risk of fibrillation, that is the torsional non-pumping mode that weak heart muscle can go into, causing death in about two minutes.

[4] To increase the elasticity of blood vessels, thereby making aneurysm of a blood vessel less likely. Aneurysm in major blood vessels can result in massive internal bleeding and in small vessels in the brain the result is haemorrhagic stroke.

[5] To reduce blood pressure.

[6] To reduce risk of osteoporosis and improve joint function.

[7] To improve bowel regularity.

[8] To reduce fatigue, stress and anxiety.

[9] Recovery from injury or surgery. It has been found, for example, that exercise programs after cancer treatments considerably increase long term survival rates.

[10] Improved physical capacity.

It has been said that the main indicator of the likelihood of a person having a heart attack is their *physical capacity,* not whether they have had a heart attack previously.

Corder (2007) also says: *"If you have already had a heart attack, daily moderate exercise is more successful than any medical treatment for preventing heart failure."*

If that isn't motivation to get a little fitter then what on earth is!

The Finnish Diabetes Prevention Study and the US Diabetes Prevention Program together involved more than 3,800 participants and showed that improved lifestyle reduced incidence of diabetes by 58% (Chris Tzar, *The Weekend Australian,* May 19-20, 2007).

The bottom line, therefore, is that a sound diet and exercise regimen will greatly reduce risk of most diseases, including cancer.

In contrast, inactivity quickly leads to musco-skeletal deterioration and skeletal muscles atrophy with the first 7 days of decreased weight bearing, whilst bone loss begins within 7 days of immobilization (Lubkin & Larsen, 2006).

Guidelines for public health developed by a group of experts commissioned by Public Health England, and published on 1 June 2015 in the British Journal of Sports Medicine recommended that workers stand for at least two hours a day, warning against the dangers of prolonged sitting.

According the Melbourne's Herald Sun on 3 June 2015:

The experts recommended people start with two hours of standing or light activity, adding that they should eventually double that to four hours.

In recent years the hazards of sitting too much have been compared to those of smoking, with research suggesting people who spend most of their days seated are more likely to be fat, have heart problems, cancer and even die earlier.

Not even regular exercise seems to help.

7. EXERCISE

The experts pointed out that those who sit the longest each day have more than double the risk of type 2 diabetes and CVD, 13% greater risk of cancer, and 17% greater risk of premature death.

A note of caution, however, for older people concerning outdoor exercise. A six-year study carried out in Sydney and published in *Osteoporosis International* in 2010 showed older people are more likely to fall and break their hip in cold weather. For those aged 75-84 fracture was 2% less likely with each 1C increase in temperature amongst men, and 1% less likely amongst women.

For those with arthritis walking might need to be limited, both in respect to speed and distance, and alternative exercises such as cycling, table tennis, and the use of 'exercise machines', including exercise bikes, might be preferred.

A recent study found that people returning to exercise too vigourously after a substantial break were likely to quickly suffer muscle damage, so that care should be taken to slowly build up intensity and duration of exercise.

Finally, note that sweating helps prevent heart disease, and a Finnish study of 2315 men aged from 42 to 60 found that those who had a sauna daily had half the risk of death from heart disease, and 40 percent lesser risk of death from any cause (Herald Sun, Melbourne, 25/2/2005).

This is because increasing sweating helps the body's lymphatic system detoxify the body to a greater extent than normal, helping eliminate excessive toxin levels (Lourie & Smith, 2013).

7. Exercise

Chapter 8

QUITTING SMOKING

> *It's easy to give up smoking, I've done it a thousand times.*
> Mark Twain.

Nicotine

Nicotine is a alkaloid, that is, a nitrogenous substance found in plants. It is absorbed by the body when tobacco is chewed or smoked causing a sympathomimetic effect in which epinephrine, a catecholamine secreted by the adrenal medulla in response to stress, stimulates autonomic nerve action. Cardiovascular symptoms of this include a rise in blood pressure and heart rate, and stimulation of the central nervous system.

As with many habituating drugs, tolerance increases and so larger doses are required with continued usage, and there are considerable psychological and physical withdrawal symptoms when usage is abruptly terminated (Morton & Hall, 1996).

Begin by cutting down

Giving up smoking, most smokers will agree, is very hard. One author on the subject makes the good point that one is really *escaping* something bad more so than giving up something good (Carr, 1999).

I would add that success is more likely if you are a little single minded and focus on quitting only one bad habit (in this case smoking) at a time. Note, however, that your 'quit plan' might involve *adding* a number of things such as improved diet and exercise.

The tobacco plant produces nicotine to poison predators and it was once used as a crop insecticide. It also kills rabbits: if you shave a patch of skin on a rabbit and paint it with nicotine it kills the rabbit.

8. Quitting Smoking

Smoking kills humans more slowly, being the main cause of lung and several other cancers.[1] It is also a major factor in atherosclerosis:

(a) By encouraging oxidation of LDL cholesterol.

(b) By causing a gene defect that triggers fibrinogen production to excess, thus encouraging growth of arterial plaques (Westcott, 2002).

One can't help but wonder why supposedly civilized people would cross the globe and, seeing savages smoking tobacco, make a point of copying them on a grand scale.

It only goes to prove that, largely thanks to that great monster Big Biz, we are deep into reverse evolution. Don't worry about Hitler and his ilk any more. Worry about what all the little Hitlers selling you harmful rubbish are doing to you to get rich very quickly.

Before I describe a suggested approach to this great problem, it seems appropriate in the context of this short book to suggest you buy a bottle of vitamin tablets if you haven't lately. If you smoke, antioxidant tablets would be appropriate as you are spending a lot of time oxidizing tobacco and sucking the resulting carcinogenic tars into your lungs.

Then note that your bottle of vitamin tablets probably cost no more than a packet of cigarettes but will last a great deal longer!

Then, if you really want to give up smoking [and you should!] the following measures are almost guaranteed to give good results:

1) Begin cutting down by not smoking during certain activities or times of the day, for example when you go out for an hour or two don't take any cigarettes (which you shouldn't have around anyway) but perhaps some chewing gum or mints instead.

As a motivation work out how much you spend on smoking in a year and then ten or twenty years, including compound interest. If you smoke much at all it should be quite a lot of money.

As another motivation note how smoking damages your lungs, impairs your breathing, increases cholesterol build up, causes loss of fitness, throat cancer, lung cancer, bladder cancer, strokes, heart attacks and countless other problems including poverty.

Evidence of such damage, a study published in JAMA in 1995 proved a relationship between smoking and inactivity, high BP, elevated cholesterol and high homocysteine levels (Cooper, 1996).

---

[1] Such as cancer of the mouth, throat, tongue, jaw, and bladder.

In addition, nicotine is a brain stimulant so the damned habit doesn't really relax you. You only feel relaxed having that next smoke because you are addicted to the stimulus it provides.

Thus a useful motivational exercise is to measure your pulse one morning and then after three of four cigarettes in an hour. Some people find an increase in pulse rate from, say, about 60 to 80. Seriously unhealthy stuff, and doing this for life will not be good for your heart and will be very bad indeed for your lungs.

2) Begin planning to use substitutes for smoking, including food, drink, chewing gum, mints, nicotine patches, a little wine, and activities including exercise, reading, writing, and games.

Note that simple food and drink are cheaper than cigarettes. In fact not paying all that tax and excise you should save heaps.

3) As preliminary exercises, try having a cup of coffee or a glass of wine without a cigarette. If you can do it once, why not always?

4) Plan the first days of giving up smoking ahead, choosing a holiday or weekend if possible so that you can get plenty of sleep to shorten the first days of abstinence. Make sure that for day 1 there are no cigarettes around and that all your substitutes are at hand.

5) On day 1 make sure you fill your diet and day with plenty of food and drink so you are at least not craving for proper sustenance.

You might immediately feel just a little too healthy so take a walk or even a bit of a run in the park and preferably nowhere near a shop that sells cigarettes. And take a pack of chewing gum instead!

6) From day 1 fill your day with plenty of activities so your mind and/or body are busy and you are not at a loose end for even a minute to get 'flashes' about getting some cigarettes

7) Don't buy any cigarettes.

8) At first, at least, avoid smokers and places where people smoke.

9) Also try and avoid stress as far as possible so you can concentrate on the main task at hand.

10) Don't restrict yourself on food or booze. Having filled your day and, if having a drink in the evening brings the thought of a cigarette, then have another sip. If you keep doing this time will pass and you will be tranquilized enough to go to bed.

Then you've made it through day 1 and the job is as good as done. Perhaps this was a day off and the next day is too, so repeat the first no smoking day exactly. After two days you have it made and should be through the physical withdrawal.

Even before day 1, having become accustomed to such things as going for a walk without taking any cigarettes and having tried such exercises as a cup of coffee without a cigarette you are well on the way.

Then on day 1 when you've gone an hour or two without a smoke you have already given it up (for a while!). Remember you also slept quite a few hours as well so should have clocked up half a day or so without a smoke. So soon as this even, you should already be feeling a little healthier without the nasty cigarettes and your lungs will already be starting to clear out thanks to small micro-organisms called biological flagella.

Note that occasional cravings for nicotine you may experience for a day or two, or even a week or two, should actually last no more than about 20 seconds and then disappear as quickly as they came.

In other words, they are simply momentary impulses and, of course, most impulses in life we have to resist, so why not smoking which is responsible for 83% of lung cancer and a third of all cancer deaths.

When you've made it to the evening you can settle down and relax, fill up on food and drink and soon go to bed. Now you really have it made and you certainly don't consider going out to buy cigarettes.

Day 2 need only copy day 1 and then you really have it done.

After day 2 you can calculate that, if you assume quitting for 100 days gives the full benefit, then after two days you get a pretty good 4% improvement! This simple calculation is given in the next section.

Needless to say, after two weeks you have it done 'with brass knobs on' and can declare openly that you've given it up.

Now you can look at other suckers who smoke with a mixture of feelings including disdain and sympathy.

Now you can also see how much money you are saving and look forward to saving heaps over the years to come.

You will also be feeling a lot healthier and can look forward to your lungs clearing out slowly over the weeks and months ahead and your lung cancer risk going back to normal over a few years.

After two weeks you definitely have it made!

If in following weeks and months you sneak just one, maybe two cigarettes somehow (don't buy any and thus have a packet to finish!) that won't matter. You should find they don't really taste too good after all.

The parabolic improvement curve

As a little psychological help, it may help to use a little *positive reinforcement* as soon as you start the quit process so think about the parabolic curve of improvement shown in Figure 8.1.

If your goal is to go 100 days without smoking (overkill - you've really largely lost the habit much sooner) then in half that time you should have three quarters of the improvement, the equation for one hundred days being:

% improvement = 100 - (1- days/100) x (100 - days)

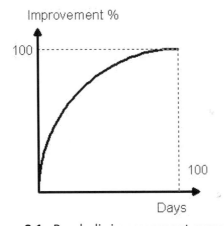

Figure 8.1. Parabolic improvement curve.

After 50 days, for example, percentile improvement is
% improvement = 100 - (1 - 50/100) x ⍰(100 - 50)
= 100 - (1/2) x (50) = 100 - 25 = 75%

After only 10 days it is
% improvement = 100 - (1 - 10/100) x⍰ (100 - 10)
= 100 - (0.9) x (90) = 100 - 81 = 19%
and even after just 2 days improvement = 4%, a worthwhile result.

To help motivate you to stick to your quit smoking program keep reminding yourself of your increasing percentile improvement with each passing day and that you don't want to sacrifice that improvement and waste all the thought and effort you may have put into quitting.

Further Motivation

No doubt you know that smoking causes lung cancer, heart disease and many other problems but it might motivate you further towards quitting to note that:

(1) A study of the records of 105,760 Swedish women found that those with high levels of HPV infection who smoked had 27 times the risk of cervical cancer compared to smokers with no HPV. In non-smokers high-level HPV infection increased risk only six-fold (*Cancer Epidemiology Biomarkers & Prevention* 15 (2005) 2141-2147).

(2) A survey of 470,000 people over 10 years published in 2011 in *the Journal of the American Medical Association* found that smokers were four times more likely to get bladder cancer.

(3) Women who smoke during pregnancy are more likely to have children with extra, webbed or missing fingers or toes (*Plastic & Reconstructive Surgery* 117 (2006) 301-308).

A study published online in *Journal of Developmental and Behavioral Pediatrics* in 2011 found that a quarter of children of women who smoked while pregnant showed a high level of delinquent behaviour.

A study of data from 19 trials published online in *Pediatrics* in 2011 found that non-smoking women exposed to second-hand smoke had a 23% greater risk of stillbirth and a 13% greater risk of congenital defects.

(4) Results of a 23-year survey of 21,000 middle-aged people published in 2011 in *Archives of Internal Medicine* showed that those who had smoked more than two packs of cigarettes a day were twice as likely to have dementia.

(5) An Australian study of 8367 sexually active men found that men who smoke 20 or more cigarettes a day are 40% more likely to suffer from impotence (*Tobacco Control* 15 (2006) 136-139).

The latter finding reminds us that smoking increases atherosclerosis by increasing oxidation of LDL cholesterol, thereby increasing risk of cardiovascular, cerebrovascular and peripheral vascular disease.

Alcohol, unless restricted to minimal 'medicinal' dosage, also contributes to vascular disease, in part simply because of the large amount of blood triglycerides that the liver struggles to convert the alcohol back into.

Both tobacco and alcohol also considerably increase the incidence of most forms of cancer.

Finally, both are expensive, particularly because of government taxes, and cost those who can least afford it a small fortune over a lifetime, in turn doing their health more damage because of the stresses of relative poverty and unhealthy lifestyle.

Conclusion

Obviously the same sort of approach applies to other drugs and other bad habits, for example:

1) Food. For the overweight, exercise, of course, is required. For specific food excesses such as chocolate the substitute is naturally healthier food with fewer calories.

2) Marihuana and other drugs. To quit much the same process as described here should work in most cases.

3) Appearance. If you are obsessed with appearance and spend a lot of time and money on cosmetics, beauty treatments, clothes and even cosmetic surgery, then substitutes might include healthy exercise or more intellectual pursuits such as study.

4) Gadgets. From PCs to cars, the substitutes might be alternative and healthier activities like exercise.

5) Games. From PC games to golf substitutes for these are simpler and more natural alternative activities without paraphernalia such as healthier activities like walking and jogging.

These are just a few examples and there are countless ways in which increasingly ubiquitous marketing brainwashes consumers into excessive consumption. A fine example of this is given in the following section.

Postscript

The sad truth is that smokers are statistically more likely to be from lower socio-economic backgrounds.

As for the idea that nicotine, a brain stimulant anyway, relaxes you, a study of 469 smokers hospitalized for heart attacks and/or surgery and who wanted to quit, published online in *Addiction* in 2010 found that a year later stress levels were lower in the 41% who had managed to quit for that year.

In fact, when people crave that next cigarette they want another stimulating 'hit' and, when not allowed it, they often go literally crazy.

As for quitting smoking, beyond the 'natural' measures suggested earlier, chewing gum containing nicotine and nicotine skin patches may be helpful (Merrell, 1995). In my view, however, ordinary chewing gum should in most cases suffice as a substitute for smoking.

Hypnosis is also claimed, by those that make money out of such claims, to help you quit cigarettes in 60 minutes. I hope that people reading this chapter two or three times and ruminating upon it for a while before devising their own quite program will get better results than they would from hypnosis. Indeed, rereading this chapter a few times might have a somewhat hypnotic effect!

Finally, Cuban health researchers have recently developed a vaccine that creates antibodies that make lung cancer tumours more manageable. As smoking is almost a tradition in Cuba, this development is being hailed as a major breakthrough.

Chapter 9

STRESS REDUCTION

- -we are very impressed with research on Transcendental Meditation
showing an 87% reduction in hospitalization for heart disease
in those who practice this technique. Add to this a 55% reduction
in hospitalizations for cancer in TM meditators.
www.alkalizeforhealth.net

Introduction

One of the most important hormones is the stress hormone adrenaline (epinephrine). Without it we might never get out of bed when the alarm rings and reminds us of our agenda for the day.

Adrenaline triggers the 'fight or flight' response and along with it:

(a) Blood vessels in the heart and brain dilate, those in the skin and gut constricting to compensate.

(b) Glucose production increases.

(c) Blood pressure, heart rate, and respiration rate increase.

(d) The lung's bronchioles are dilated.

(3) As a protective mechanism in case of injury the blood is enriched with platelets that help clotting.

Little wonder that, with all this going on, stress can cause angina or a heart attack, particularly if the coronary arteries are significantly occluded by cholesterol plaques.

Perhaps more important in the longer term, synthesis of adrenalin requires vitamin C so that prolonged stress can deplete vitamin C levels, rendering arteries, especially those in the heart, more prone to deterioration and thus atherosclerosis (Rath 2001b).[1]

---

[1] See chapter 2 for an introduction to the 'vitamin C theory' of heart disease.

9. STRESS REDUCTION

The *Lancet* reported a study in which the ECG readings of 14 heart patients indicated insufficient oxygen or *ischemia* when they were performing simple arithmetic tests. Similarly raised cholesterol levels have been found in students before exams.

Nursing manuals describe two types of heart patients, types A and B. Type A's are impatient, fussy, goal-oriented with tunnel vision and stress both themselves and those around them. Type B's are not.

A 15 year study of 2105 healthy Vietnam veterans found that "negative" personality traits such as depression, anxiety, hostility and anger increased the heart disease risk factors of high cholesterol, high blood pressure and high body mass index (*Psychosomatic Med* V 10, 2006, p 1087).

A 37-year study of 50,000 men published in 2010 found that those who had been anxious at 18-20 were more than twice as likely to develop cardiovascular disease or have a heart attack (*J Am Coll Cardiol* 2010; 56; 31-37).

Recent research at John Hopkins University indicated that people with 'hot' reactions who scored high in 'mental stress' tests were more than 20 times more likely to develop cardiovascular disease.

It has recently been found that C-reactive protein levels, a marker for cardiovascular disease, were as high in men with trait-anger as they were in those who were obese or smoked. This led to the conclusion that anger management might have more than just psychological benefits.

If follows that stress management may have physiological benefits.

Besides the ongoing stresses of day-to-day life there are the ongoing stresses that result from major personal disasters such as loss of a job or spouse. An example of the latter is that the immune systems of widows and widowers have been found to be impaired for more than a year.

Indeed, women are more than twice as likely to die after the death of a spouse, and men more than six times, a phenomenon called *broken heart syndrome*. This is thought to be caused by dysfunctional microvasculature, sometimes resulting in heart attacks in people with normal coronary arteries.

Similarly, demographic studies have found a much increased incidence of severe or fatal heart attacks after major earthquakes.

There is much evidence that children are likely to benefit if parents de-stress and cheer up, for example:

(1) Decades of research has shown that about half the children of depressed mothers develop depression, three times the normal incidence (*The Weekend Australia*, May 21-22, 2011).

(2) A study published in *The American Journal of Psychiatry* in 2011 also found that children of depressed mothers are more likely to be anxious, irritable and disruptive.

(3) A study published in 2011 in *Pediatrics* found that depressed fathers were half as likely to read to their children but four times more likely to spank them.

Techniques for dealing with everyday stress

Some examples of strategies for dealing with day to day stress:

[1] Learn to recognize conditions that stress you and convince yourself that these situations are best dealt with calmly.

[2] Remember Mohr's First Law of War: *Don't Panic.*

[3] Work out how to prevent or avoid stressful situations.

[4] Make sure you have somebody to talk to when things go wrong.

[5] Cultivate the habit of taking time out to quietly reflect on, rationalize, and come to terms with adverse events.

[6] Try and reorganize events that you find annoying so that they are more to your satisfaction. For example, if possible change venues and timing for meetings you find stressful.

[7] If certain people annoy you try and stand above it. Consider their actions a sign of weakness, allowing you to feel the master of the situation, even in dealing with your boss.

[8] Talk to people who annoy you rather than holding a grudge. They may quickly see your point of view and even apologize for annoying you!

[9] Eat well. A satisfied tummy has a calming effect in great contrast to that of being even a bit behind on calorie intake for the day.

[10] Sleep well. There is no doubt that a fair amount of good quality sleep will be beneficial to your health and help you cope with life better.

The bottom line here is tackle problems, and indeed life itself, more carefully and thoughtfully.

Relaxation techniques

There are a number of techniques for stress reduction that may be used in alternation or a favourite one chosen.

For each of these: (a) Find 30 minutes daily to yourself, away from noise and other distractions.

(b) Make yourself comfortable and dim the lights.

(c) If your mind wanders or is distracted, simply focus again on the technique you are using. Aim for increasing calmness and relaxation.

[1] Muscle relaxation

Seated or lying down, imagine your body floating and mentally focus on each muscle group in turn. Contract the muscles for 10 seconds and then relax them consciously for 10 seconds.

[2] Yoga

Yoga is a series of poses that stretch different muscle groups. It is easiest to devise your own poses that you can do comfortably and hold for 20 seconds, meditating at the same time.

Imagine your mind leaving your body [this is serious! - if you can't take it seriously remember that laughter is supposed to be good for the heart].

[3] Breathing meditation

Close your eyes and concentrate on each breath. If you are an ex-smoker it might help to notice how much more relaxing it is without nicotine, an addictive stimulant.

Start by doing this for 5 or 10 minutes and gradually increase the time to 30 minutes. Your mind may wander to life's problems much of the time but simply refocus on your breathing as much as possible.

[4] Mindfulness meditation

Begin with a few minutes of breathing meditation and then concentrate upon feeling detached as though observing things from on high. Then quietly view your thoughts or any other stimuli that present themselves without judgment or feelings.

It is common for suppressed or repressed memories to be recalled. If these are disturbing they are best forgotten by changing to some physical rather than meditation relaxation technique.

On the other hand, you might revive some good memories that put you in a more positive frame of mind for the rest of the day.

[5] Self-hypnosis

Begin with a brief body scan (as in [1]) for a few minutes. Close your eyes, relax, and visualize yourself in a time machine. The time machine is gradually moving backwards and you see happy scenes of people at work and play in the sun with views of beaches, fields, forests, rivers and mountains.

Move your mind to a beach on a tropical island. Hear the warm azure blue waves gently caressing your toes and feel the warmth of the sun on your body. You are half-asleep and your mind is floating a few feet above you in a pleasant daze.

[6] Music

Quiet, soothing music without lyrics helps with relaxation and might accompany any of the foregoing relaxation methods.

[7] Exercise

Exercise such as walking in pleasant surroundings can, of course, be used to reduce stress. Many athletes say that they get a lift out of exercising. This is because of beta-endormorphins released into the blood during vigourous exercise. In taking a walk for relaxation purposes we want just the opposite to happen - not a 'buzz' of excitement - but a feeling of calmness sweeping over us.

[8] Eye exercises

Eye exercises can help correct vision problems that arise with aging such as myopia (short-sightedness) and hyperopia (long-sightedness). These can be done while relaxing in the evenings, examples being:

(a) Close one eye and imagine you are looking at a pinhead at the centre of a photograph in a magazine, thus giving a slightly 3-D view, a phenomenon called monocular stereoscopy. Practicing this with both eyes improves 'visual depth perception' (Brookes-Simpkins, 1968).

(b) Hold one end of a piece of string to the tip of your nose with the tip of a finger and gradually stretch the string as far as you can straight out in front of you with the other hand, letting your focus follow your moving hand and the sharp end of the illusion of two strings in a 'Vee' shape that you see.

Two or three minutes of these simple exercises daily will help maintain proper function of the eye muscles and help avert, or at least reduce, the need for glasses.

To protect your eyes you should also ensure that they are protected from glare by, for example, ensuring that light bulb filaments are not directly visible. Wearing sunglasses out of doors, of course, is mandatory.

To relax your eyes it is useful to have muted and relaxing 'background' lighting in the home. It is also helpful if this is in 'relaxing' hues such as green and, indeed, it has been suggested that 'visible ray therapy' using different colours might be a way of curing many eye afflictions ranging from glaucoma to cataracts (Brookes-Simpkins, 1968).

[9] Sleep

Sleep is a way to de-stress as long as you sleep soundly. A large long-term study published in 2010 found that children aged 2-4 who had sleeping problems were more likely to have attention problems when they were 14. The moral would appear to be that if you are less stressed you should sleep better, good sleep probably de-stressing you further.

Styling your life to reduce stress

Ways in which you can reduce stress in your life include:

[1] Social networks

Going out and socializing can also take your mind off things. Friends can be useful for advice and support whereas bottling up problems can more than double risk of heart disease in men (*J Epidemiology and Community Heath*, 2011;65;420-425)

[2] Rest and recreation

Make sure you get plenty of recreation and include plenty of exercise in this. Make sure too that you get enough sleep, if not a little extra.

[3] Financial management

Unless you really do have too much money, don't spend money on unnecessary things that you don't need and don't get into debt needlessly.

All this is easier said than done in a marriage with children and a mortgage, when the odds are that both partners have their little extravagances and that one of the two is not very good with money.

[4] Actively deal with problems

A 10-year study of 2755 men found that those who coped covertly with unfair treatment at work had 2.3 times the risk of heart attack or death from heart disease than those who dealt with the issue in other ways (Leinweber et al., 2009).

[5] Lifelong learning

Statistics show that better educated people live a little longer, no doubt in part thanks to higher income and greater job satisfaction.

Thus, habits and interests like reading, music, writing, painting, bush walking and the like will help keep you happier and younger.

[6] Dealing with emotional traumas

When major crises like death in the family, accidents or job problems are getting you down make sure you have somebody constructive to talk to. Sometimes you will find professionals are better listeners than friends and more likely to propose ways of coping.

[7] Depression

Solitude can be depressing. Statistics show that married men live longer than single ones and men that have never been married fare worst on this score.

Women around 30-40 who have never been married or had children may experience depression, the term *hysteria* being used in psychiatry in part because its meaning in ancient Greek was 'without a womb' and the term was applied to childless women.

[8] Alcohol and other drugs

Nicotine is a brain stimulant so it doesn't relax you. Quite on the contrary, you get hooked so that having another dose of stimulant simply restores the bad status quo of higher pulse rate and blood pressure, just signs of the damage being done inside.

The same sort of thing applies to other drugs.

Alcohol deserves special mention as it is a drug which has a great hold on (Western) society in which many people are addicted to it.

Decades ago a 7 year US study of 11,000 middle-aged men found that those who had two standard drinks a day had higher HDL than those who didn't. They also had a 22% reduction in fatal heart disease.

It was concluded that HDL increase was because of stress reduction effects, not because of the alcohol. A 1984 study found that alcohol had no effect on HDL in people who undertook regular aerobic exercise.

We've all heard many stories of centenarians swearing by their daily drink or two. These suggest that such people are careful in everything, including their diet, and that is responsible for their longevity.

Conclusions

We've already mentioned Mohr's First Law of War, namely *Don't Panic*. The second is *Be Prepared* because there is nothing like the panic of finding that you've forgotten to bring the essential item when it's time to do something.

In other words, take time out to relax, rest, and think a bit. Then you can devise solutions to your problems, perhaps with the help of others.

A study of 15,000 heart attacks in 52 countries published in *The Lancet* found that stress is responsible for more than a fifth of heart attacks worldwide (reported in *The Weekend Australian,* Sept. 4-5, 2004).

This was backed up by a 10-year study of 1700 people published in the *European Heart Journal* which found that people with a positive outlook had 25% lesser risk of heart disease.

Furthermore, it has been found in clinical trials that people at risk of heart attack have been able to reduce their risk of an attack as much by stress reduction techniques as by exercise, both measures proving as beneficial, if not more so, than medication.

The placebo affect can also alleviate heart pain. Ogden cites a study in which half a group of heart patients were given a bypass operation and half a "sham operation", both groups having an equal reduction in pain (Ogden, 2007).

Notably, researchers have found that stress during pregnancy can affect a baby's development in the womb, artificially boosted levels of a natural stress hormone in pregnant mice causing them to eat more, reducing transport of glucose to the foetus and modifying some genes in the placenta adversely (Herald Sun, Melbourne, 25/1/2015).

In meditation or even in sleep you might find some answers. If you wake during the first couple of REM sleep periods that happen every 90 minutes or so you might find you are having a bad dream. If you wake in the second last REM period you will often find that your brain gives you an idea on some current problem (Brookes-Simpkins, 1968). If you wake during the last REM period before the time the alarm is set for you may well find yourself thinking of the key thing you have to do today!

Another motive for meditation is that mindfulness meditation has been found to increase brain size. A 2009 UCLA study published in 2009 used MRI to show that long-term meditators had larger volumes of regions of the brain which regulate emotions, namely the hippocampus and orbitofrontal cortex, the thalamus, and the inferior temporal gyrus.

US expert on meditation Thom Knoles says:

"Practicing meditation helps us see things clearly, have a stronger sense of self and puts the stresses in our lives into proper perspective.

Research indicates that the effects of meditation are not just that the brain is growing more grey matter, but that the brain is learning how to repair itself organically. It would not be out of the question to assume that the brain is actually regenerating cells" (*The Sunday Herald Sun*, Melbourne, July 3, 2011).

Now that is surely motivation for meditation.

Finally, note that magnesium helps counter stress, firstly by being crucial to muscle relaxation so that it dilates arteries and is thus very helpful in treating variant angina, as noted in later chapters.

Secondly, magnesium helps the body counter stress hormones so that they do not effect stress levels as much.

Indeed, current studies suggest that chronic stress reduces immune system function, increasing cancer risk, raising the possibility of using beta blockers to prevent the spread of breast cancer (Nick Toscano, 'Stress test: cancer link', *Wyndam Weekly*, 12/9/2012). Magnesium is often found more effective than beta blockers in the treatment of variant angina and thus should also be effective in reducing the cancer-encouraging effects of stress.

Finally, note that:

(a) Lack of sleep decreases release of the 'feel-good' chemical dopamine and other hormones, increasing the likelihood of addiction to *"simple carbohydrates and sugars as well as the aging fats that are the imposters to real food"* (Roizen & Mehmet, 2005).

(b) Sometimes dieting can increase levels of stress hormones but stress reduction techniques can alleviate this problem (Turner, 2009).

(c) Stress reduction techniques can, of course, reduce anxiety levels and depression, as can exercise (Minirth & Meier, 2007).

(d) A one-hour daytime nap was found to lower blood pressure by 4 percent during the day, and by 6 per cent when sleeping at night.

(e) A study of 4,000 people of average age 75 found that those with lower level thinking skills were 85 per cent more likely to have a heart attack, and 51 per cent more likely to have a stroke, showing that heart and brain function are closely related.

9. Stress Reduction

Chapter 10

ALCOHOL IN MODERATION

> *Truth be told, however, heavier alcohol consumption provides other*
> *protective benefits against heart disease.*
> *Almost grudgingly, a commentary in the British medical journal*
> *'The Lancet' in 2005 pointed out that during autopsies,*
> *the coronary arteries of alcoholics are frequently relatively 'clean',*
> *indicating a linear level of protection, whether from elevated*
> *HDL cholesterol, reduced levels of inflammation, or whatever.*
> Robert E Kowalski, *Take The Pressure Off Your Heart* (2006).

Moderate alcohol intake reduces mortality

The alcohol issue is an interesting one. In the 19th century snake oil salesmen sang the praises of their product. Today we hear publicity about the virtues of most food products and bad publicity about having too much saturated fat, salt or alcohol and little else.

Recently there have been meat industry sponsored TV ads in Australia imploring us to eat red meat 3 times a week which flies in the face of the current wisdom that it is fish that we should be aiming to eat 3 times a week. When we hear of French studies that find red wine is beneficial, therefore, we might be a little sceptical.

Some experts recommend half to one standard drink (SD) a day for women and one to two a day for men for heart health because:

(a) The Nurses Health Study of nearly 90,000 nurses in the USA found that those who had 3 or more drinks a week had 40% fewer fatal heart attacks (Roizen, 2000).

(b) A long-term study of 8867 healthy men with a healthy lifestyle found that over the period from 1986 to 2002 those who had an average of two standard drinks a day suffered 62% fewer heart attacks than those who abstained from alcohol (K Mukamal et al., *Arch Intern Med* 166 (2006) 2145-2150).

(c) A Dutch study of more than 50,000 people reported in *The Weekend Australian* (27-28 May 2006) found that men who drank moderately only once a week had only a 7% reduction in risk of heart disease whereas those who drank daily had a 41% risk reduction.

In contrast, women who drank weekly had a 35% risk reduction and those who drank daily had a 36% risk reduction.

For men at least, it appears that a daily tipple is the most beneficial. This is as one might expect if one compared the practice of a daily drink or two to that of taking half an aspirin once or twice daily, obligatory for those with heart attack or stroke risk.

The positive effects of alcohol in moderation

The reasons that a daily tipple might be beneficial to the high risk groups of middle-aged men and post-menopausal women include:

(1) It is well known that regular moderate alcohol consumption increases HDL levels slightly, but not the heart protective HDL2b mainly responsible for reverse cholesterol transport (Superko, 2004). In any event, exercise is a more effective way of increasing HDL levels (Cooper, 1996) but this may not be an option for the very ill.

(2) A study of 2000 Germans found that moderate drinkers had lower levels of C-reactive protein (CRP), an *acute phase reactant*, a protein released rapidly into the bloodstream to tackle inflammation. As a result they had fewer signs of inflammation in the body compared to nondrinkers or heavy drinkers (Cooke and Zimmer, 2002). CRP is a marker for inflammation and high levels of CRP are twice as likely to be a precursor to heart attack than high LDL-C (Superko, 2004).

Note that fish oils and aspirin also reduce inflammation.

(3) Alcohol is a tranquilizer and, as such, it is a vasodilator. Alcohol's vasodilatory effect can be graphically demonstrated by shining a light through a rabbit's ears and then injecting it with a little alcohol after which further inspection shows up small capillaries that were not visible before. This effect, however, is only a short-term one.

(4) Most wines are made from vitis vinifera grape varieties and the malic acid in these has been claimed to reduce atherosclerotic plaques and is used together with EDTA (see Chapter 2) and garlic to 'chelate' calcium from plaques (www.arteryhealthinstitute.com).

The benefits of red wine

(1) Scientist Serge Renaud tracked 34,000 Frenchmen, 75% of whom drank red wine, for 15 years and found those who had 2-3 glasses daily had a 30% lesser death rate and were 35% less likely to die of heart disease and 18-24% less likely to die of cancer (Carper, 2000). The reduction in cancer death rates was presumably because of the renowned antioxidant properties of red wine.

(2) Small amounts of the substance endothelin-1 are needed to maintain the structural integrity of blood vessels but excessive amounts cause arterial constriction, hardening, and ultimately atherosclerosis.

Unhealthy arteries have increased endothelin-1 and reduced production of nitric oxide (NO), the endothelial-derived relaxation factor (EDRF), a vasodilator. The polyphenols, particularly the procyanidins, in red wine are able to restore healthy endothelial function, in part by increasing production of NO (Corder, 2007). White wine does not have this beneficial function to any extent.

Other antioxidants in red wine such as resveratrol and quercetin also protect NO (nitric oxide) and thus relax blood vessels (Cooke and Zimmer, 2002), but "many red wines have a high procyanidin content, with amounts close to 1g per litre, which is around a thousand times the average level of resveratrol" (Corder, 2007).

(3) Alcohol is an anticoagulant which reduces platelet aggregation and thus thins the blood because it increases TPA or tissue plasminogen activator (McGowan, 1998). A US study found that 2.5 glasses of red wine reduced blood stickiness by 40% within 45 minutes (Carper, 2000).

A French study with animals showed that blood-clotting activity (platelet stickiness or aggregation) was initially depressed by red wine, white wine and straight alcohol. 14 hours later red wine had kept blood stickiness down by 60% but with white wine it had rebounded to be 46% higher (than normal) and with plain alcohol it was a huge 124% higher.

In another study, however, synthetic wine increased platelet clumping, white wine made no difference, and red wine decreased platelet clumping (Carper, 2000).

(4) The antioxidants in red wine reduce oxidation of LDL and deposition of the resulting material in the artery walls, the primary stage of atherosclerosis (Cooke and Zimmer, 2002).

The J-curve for alcohol

Some people find that the 'safe' 4 glasses of wine in one sitting tends to affect their stomach lining a little even if consumed very slowly, a reminder that alcohol does cause ulcers and cancer all the way through the digestive system and elsewhere. Larger doses might produce what Carper (2000) refers to as "holiday heart syndrome," that is people suffering severe arrhythmia after weekend or holiday binges, particularly between Christmas Eve and New Year's Day. Thus, binge drinkers have been found twice as likely as moderate drinkers to get heart disease

Withdrawal effects after a binge include reversal of both blood thinning and arterial dilation which are likely to cause BP to rise sharply to dangerous levels, increasing the risk of an aneurysm in the heart or brain 'blowing', presumably one reason why one study found that 40% of women who died suddenly were diagnosed alcoholics (Carper, 2000)

As Kowalski (2006) points out, taking the ill-effects of excessive alcohol consumption, such as increased liver damage and cancer risk, into account, the nett benefits of alcohol follow a J-curve with increasing consumption, and one study found that heart muscle damage generally occurs with 5 or more drinks a day (Corder, 2007).

One reason for care with alcohol is clear to those having practiced home brewing. About 40 gm of refined sugar is added to make a 750 ml bottle of beer, quite a lot of sugar and, of course, our liver breaks down the alcohol so its long-run effect is similar to that of sugar. This is why "a single alcoholic drink can raise triglyceride levels" (McGowan, 1998) and, like LDL, triglycerides play a major role in atherosclerosis.

In a 1994 study 3 glasses of red wine daily increased triglyceride levels by 11% after one week, and by 26% after two weeks (Cooper, 1996). The situation is worse with white wine, beer or spirits and just 4 - 5 drinks per week can raise triglyceride levels substantially in some people (Superko, 2004). This is one of the main reasons for the J-curve regarding the benefits of alcohol.

Evidence of this, two studies published online in *The British Medical Journal* in 2011 found that light drinking reduced risk of heart disease and stroke and death from these. One study found that the lowest risk of death from heart disease was with 1-2 drinks a day. The other found moderate drinking improved blood markers for heart disease.

Recommendations on dosage

Numerous studies suggest that 'moderate' alcohol consumption gives significant heart protection and most writers agree that at least somewhere from 1 - 4 standard drinks (SD) a day is safe and beneficial and more than this does more harm than good.

Table 10.1. Australian alcohol guidelines (2006).

SD/day	Safe	Risky	High Risk
Men, long term	≤ 4	5 - 6	> 6
Men, short term	≤ 6 on ≤ 3 days of week	7 - 10 on one day of week	>10 on one day of week
Women, long term	≤ 2	3 - 4	> 4
Women, short term	≤ 4 on ≤ 3 days of week	5 - 6 on one day of week	> 6 on one day of week

Table 10.1 shows the previous NHMRC Australian Alcohol Guidelines, suggesting 2 standard drinks (SD) daily for women and 4 for men as "safe" in the long term. These recommendations still make sense for those with heart disease or congestive stroke in mind, but when overall risk of death from all causes, including accident, is considered, only 1 or 2 standard drinks is associated with reduced mortality rate. Thus the tighter current guidelines are:

(1) No more than 2 SD/day for "healthy men and women."

(2) No more than 4 SD on a single occasion to reduce "risk of alcohol-related injury."

Recommendation (1) is based on the results of Table 10.2 (NHMRC, 2009b; Corrao et al., 1999).

US recommendations are sometimes more cautious and, whilst most US authors recommend only 'one or two' daily, some are more cautious and suggest just one a day, if that (Cooper, 1996; McGowan, 1998).

One factor likely to bias statistical findings, however, is that people who are careful enough to have just one drink a day are almost certain to be careful with everything else, and especially diet. One might expect, therefore, that statistically they would indeed have far lesser risk of death from all causes. In other words, the health benefits of minimal to moderate alcohol consumption may tend to be overestimated.

Table 10.2. Risks of alcohol-related death vs SD daily.

SD/day	Men			Women		
	Injury	Disease	Total	Injury	Disease	Total
1	0.20	0.21	0.41	0.13	0.16	0.29
2	0.48	0.44	0.92	0.39	0.38	0.77
3	1.50	1.26	2.76	0.91	1.41	2.32
4	2.21	1.99	4.20	1.32	2.53	3.85
5	3.11	2.70	5.81	1.84	3.68	5.52
6	5.29	3.80	9.09	2.99	5.93	8.92
7	7.51	4.66	12.17	4.16	7.61	11.77
8	9.69	5.14	14.83	5.33	8.37	13.70

It should also be noted that very few people will really have just a drink or two day in and day out, and never more than that. In reality they will 'sometimes', at least, have 'a few'. Here 'sometimes' might be once a week, once a month, or once in a blue moon. A 'few' might be a bottle of favourite wine, a six-pack of beer, or just a few extra glasses from a decanter on the sideboard.

Indeed, it might be quite likely that this practice is beneficial and could be one reason why so many large studies find that 'moderate' alcohol consumption over the long term reduces heart disease and stroke.

In contrast, a University College of London study found that when "average drinkers" abstained for a month their liver function and blood pressure and cholesterol levels improved, emphasizing that over the longer term alcohol consumption should be kept low.

The therapeutic dose

The Australian Alcohol Guidelines 2006 do allow the possible 'few' of up to 6 for ladies, and 10 for men, respectively quite close to a bottle of wine or a six-pack of beer. Such a 'therapeutic dose' involving just a couple of extra drinks is fine for that special occasion, as a treat, or just to relax, especially if it is red wine rich in procyanidins.

The Preface refers to heart pain and TIA episodes experienced by the author quite early in life. About 15 percent of major strokes are preceded by TIAs days, weeks, or months earlier (Donatalle, 2011), but fortunately the author has not had a noticeable TIA for 20+ years.

On a couple of occasions in recent years his clogged left coronary artery became quite painful after intense evening writing efforts in bad posture with a PC on a coffee table.

On one occasion the pains persisted for four days so he canceled his evening writing session and had half a dozen glasses of port and a couple of aspirin over a period of five hours. By the end of an evening in which it had crossed his mind to consider going to hospital the problem was gone!

Finally, in defence of a little too much sometimes, despite the risks, a 2005 article in *The Lancet* notes that autopsies often find the coronary arteries of alcoholics to be relatively "clean" (Kowalski, 2006).

In addition, a survey of 3052 people, 1648 of whom had been diagnosed with rheumatoid arthritis, published in *Annals of the Rheumatic Diseases* in 2007, indicated that people with the highest alcohol consumption were 40 - 50% less likely to develop the disease.

Alternatives

Red wine in moderation is beneficial because it is relatively high in antioxidants, particularly procyanidins. There are, however, plenty of other sources of similar benefits, for example:

(1) Purple grape juice has the same antioxidant and anticoagulant, benefits as red wine but only to about half the same extent. Concord purple grape juice (from the northern USA), however, has greater concentrations of some red grape antioxidants than red wines and is said to be comparable to aspirin as a clot buster and have cancer protective effects (Cooper, 1996; www.welchs.com).

In one study, patients with coronary heart disease who drank about 320 ml of Concord grape juice twice a day for two weeks had improved endothelium-dependent vasodilation.

In another study, endothelium-dependent vasodilation was obtained with red wine and dealcoholized red wine, the latter being more active than the red wine, whereas a vodka drink had no effect (Corder, 2007).

(2) Cocoa also contains procyanidins and in one study patients consuming dark chocolate for 15 days had reduced blood pressure, LDL cholesterol and insulin sensitivity (Corder, 2007).

Once again, moderation is the key as only 20 - 30 gm of procyanidin-rich dark chocolate is required to be beneficial, whereas much more than this will involve too many calories (Corder, 2007).

(3) Apples and cranberries are also rich in procyanidins whilst raspberries, strawberries, red currants and pomegranates contain polyphenols with similar benefits to procyanidins (Corder, 2007).

(4) Pinto beans, sorghum grain and cinnamon are also good sources of procyanidins.

(5) 40 grams of walnuts contains a comparable amount of polyphenols to 125 ml of red wine and a Spanish study found that a Mediterranean diet plus 40 - 65 gm of walnuts daily improved endothelium-dependent vasodilation and reduced LDL-C by 64% (Corder, 2007).

(6) Pomegranate juice has more antioxidant effect than red wine or green tea, almost halving LDL oxidation and reducing atherogenesis (BBC news online, 28/11/2004), some studies finding that it may even reverse atherosclerosis (WebMD Health News 21/3/05).

Others studies indicate that it reduces BP (in just 2 weeks), inhibits prostate, breast, lung and skin cancer, inhibits osteoarthritis, inhibits brain deterioration, and has antiviral and antibacterial properties (thus reducing periodontitis) [Wikipedia, healthdiaries.com/eatthis/, suite101.com].

(7) 1000 mg of Vitamin C has more blood antioxidant effect than 300 ml of wine: +22% after 1 hour and + 29% after 2 hours, compared to +18%/+11% for red wine and +4%/+7% for white wine (Cooper, 1996).

Red wine, however, has different antioxidants and it is best to take a range of antioxidants because, for example, vitamins C and E are synergistic in cancer protection because C is water-soluble and protects cells and E is fat-soluble and protects cell membranes.

(8) The beneficial effects of pycnogenol, a patented proprietary product, are ascribed to the antioxidant activity of procyanidins and are claimed as many, including:

➢ Improved endothelial function and lower BP.
➢ Lesser risk of heart disease and cancer.
➢ Prevention of blood clots and deep vein thrombosis (DVT).
➢ Anti-inflammatory effects and reduced arthritis symptoms.
➢ Helpful with asthma and chronic bronchitis.
➢ Protection against eye diseases and sight loss (Corder, 2007).

(9) Hawthorn extract, a popular herbal remedy for heart disease, is rich in procyanidins and clinical studies have shown improved cardiac function, greater exercise tolerance and decrease in heart-failure related symptoms (Corder, 2007).

Don't forget aspirin

The Nurses' Health Study of almost 90,000 nurses found those who took low to moderate doses of aspirin (1- 14 tablets per week) for the long term had 38% lower risk of death from heart disease, 12 % lower risk of death from cancer, and 25% lower risk of death from all causes (*Arch Int Med* 167 (2007) 562-572). Using aspirin for 1 - 6 years reduces heart risk, but cancer risk was only reduced after 10 years of aspirin use.

Another well-controlled study found that taking aspirin daily reduced heart attack incidence by 44% by making platelets less sticky and decreasing arterial inflammation (Roizen & Mehmet, 2005).

The author, therefore, has half an aspirin after breakfast as a precaution against possible ill-effects from 'morning surge', the higher BP that we all experience after lying prone to sleep for a substantial period and then suddenly arising (Kowalski, 2006).

Conclusion

Presently The World Health Organization recommends "low to moderate alcohol consumption to reduce coronary artery disease" (Wikipedia, *'coronary artery disease'*, August 2009).

Circa 2 wines a day decreases death risk by 30%, heart risk by 30 to 40% and stroke risk by 45% (Carper, 2000) but >1 beer a day increases stroke risk by 9% (Carper, 2000) and >3 beers a day increases likelihood of high BP threefold (Kowalski, 2006).

As for the much referred to 'French Paradox', surely the most careful Frenchman sometimes quietly finishes his bottle of red wine in one evening and that, done occasionally this extra couple of drinks might increase longevity, but note that this would not apply if he were drinking acidic 'rotgut' wine that one feels burning the throat etc. after a few.

If so, this must be because this slightly higher level of dosage thins the blood and expands the arteries enough to help clear them. This might be analogous to the way in which, to be really effective, exercise must involve various levels of intensity.

Equally, it is likely that the long-living people of south-west France who drink procyanidin-rich wine with their meals see no reason not to do this daily so that the daily 'medicinal dose' does seem to be the best practice (Corder, 2007). An example of this, a 15 year study of 12,000 people aged 65-75 published online in *Addiction* in 2010 found that up to 4 standard drinks a day for men and 2 for women reduced risk of death.

Aspirin, is also an anti-inflammatory agent as well as a clot buster, and can be used in conjunction with dark grape juice to obtain the same effects as red wine. As with antioxidants, however, it is probably best to hedge one's bets and have both red wine and aspirin, hoping for slightly different and perhaps complementary or synergistic effects.

As a bottom line, therefore, the daily 'medicinal' dose of a couple of drinks is desirable but it is difficult to believe that this alone is responsible for the high reduction in heart statistics attributed to it.

It might be wise to also have:

(a) Half an aspirin once or twice daily.

(b) An occasional 'therapeutic' dose of alcohol, that is a couple of drinks more than usual, with the proviso that one keeps one's average daily intake at the usual 'medicinal' level. Preferably, the extra calories are worked off with exercise.

(c) A sound diet and exercise routine.

For quenching one's thirst throughout the day the alternatives are many, including tea, coffee, cocoa, and fruit or vegetable juice of which there are many very tasty combinations available these days.

In moderation caffeine is beneficial. A study of of 6594 people aged between 32 and 86 with no history of heart disease found those aged 65 or older who drank four or more caffeinated drinks daily had a 53% lower risk of death from heart disease than those who drank less than half a caffeinated drink per day. Caffeine was found not to protect those under age 65 or those with high blood pressure (JA Greenberg at al., *Am J Clinical Nutrition* 85 (2007) 392-398). Another study found that those who drank 3-5 coffees daily were less likely to have clogged and calcified arteries (Herald-Sun, 4/3/2015).

Tea also contains polyphenols, green tea having twice as much of these as black tea. Tea improves endothelial function in patients with heart disease, a number of studies finding that drinking 3 cups of tea daily reduced heart disease by an average of 11% (Corder, 2007).

Finally, note that the amount of beneficial procyanidins in red wines varies greatly. For example, just a small glass of Madiran, a red wine made in the south-west of France, "can provide more benefit than two bottles of most Australian wine" (Corder, 2007) and contains 3-4 times more procyanidins than procyanidin-rich Argentinian Cabernet Sauvignon.

In Australia, Cabernet Sauvigons from a few smaller wineries have the highest procyanidin content (Corder, 2007).

10. ALCOHOL IN MODERATION

Cautionary note: Infected and bad tasting wines, and even good but dry and acidic to the throat wines, may contain deleterious substances such as *methyl alcohol*, CH_3OH, which is poisonous and perhaps carcinogenic, and ethylene glycol or *formalin*, $CH_2(OH)_2$ [formaldehyde in aqueous solution, formaldehyde being formed by oxidation of methyl alcohol], which hardens proteins and is used in embalming and to preserve biological specimens. That bottom line is that alcohol is a poison which in substantial doses does great harm to the brain, the digestive tract, the lungs, the liver, the spleen and the bowel. In modest doses, however, like aspirin, it is beneficial, particularly in relation to heart disease, as the results of Table 10.2 show.

Another negative property of alcohol is that its energy value is nearly 7 calories per gram, whereas the values for carbohydrate, protein and fat are respectively 4.2, 4.3 and 9.4 (Schmidt-Nielson, 1979). Thus, those concerned about losing weight should restrict both alcohol and fat intake.

The procyanidins in red wine are particularly beneficial.

It is interesting to note that another cyanide-related compound, amygdalin or vitamin B17, has been found effective in treating cancer (Mohr, 2012b, 2013).

Finally, note that Corder (2007) found that men in the South of France live about 5 years longer than those in the North, and believed this may have been because of reduced incidence of heart disease thanks to the high procyanidin content of the red wines in the South of France.

I believe that other reasons for this greater longevity might have been reduced aging and cancer incidence thanks to higher procyanidin intake, as well as better climate.

To minimize cancer risk one should have red wines with circa 10% alcohol content, not the heavier reds with up to 14% even a couple of glasses of which will begin to irritate the digestive and respiratory tract, an extreme example being alcoholic lung damage with high and prolonged alcohol intake.

Spirits with circa 40+% alcohol content should be avoided, of course, and having ice with them to reduce 'burning' sensations may not reduce the damage much.

Finally, note that excessive alcohol consumption causes cardiomyopathy (weakened heart muscles), one symptom of which may be low blood pressure.

10. Alcohol in Moderation

Chapter 11

FATS AND CHOLESTEROL

> The study shows people with high blood cholesterol face
> a 3.25 times higher risk of a heart attack or stroke
> than those with normal levels.
> Report of article in *The Lancet* published
> in *The Weekend Australian,* Sept. 4-5, 2004.

Fatty acids

The fatty acids are also known as the carboxylic acids because they contain the carboxylic group COOH. They are one of a number of groups of organic compounds, others being alcohols, amines and hydrocarbons.

The group includes the saturated (hydrogenated) straight-chain acids which have a single carboxyl group and are produced by hydrolysis, a double decomposition reaction of a compound AB with water of the form

$$AB + HOH \rightarrow AH + BOH$$

The fatty acids group also includes saturated acids with branched chain or cyclic structures. The simplest fatty acids are formic acid, HCOOH, and acetic acid, CH_3COOH, the major precursor to the 36-step reaction that produces cholesterol in the body. Both have a sharp smell while more complex structured butyric, caproic and caprylic acids all have unpleasant odors.

Stearic, palmitic, oleic, and napthenic acids are greasy materials with little odor. Fatty acids have many commercial uses, including in the manufacture of detergents, paint thickeners, lubricants, rubber, and plastics. Stearic acid, $CH_3(CH_2)_{16}COOH$, comes from many animal and vegetable fats. It gets its name from the Greek word for tallow and has many uses. It is a waxy solid that melts at 70 °C and it is a constituent of many saturated fats.

The alcohols

The simplest alcohol is methyl alcohol or methanol, CH_3OH, sometimes called wood alcohol because it was originally made from 'destructive distillation' of wood. Ethyl alcohol or ethanol, C_2H_5OH, is sometimes called grain alcohol because it has been produced by fermentation of grains since 3,000 B.C.

Ethanol is produced by the reaction of simple sugars with the yeast enzyme zymase. For glucose the reaction is:

$$C_6H_{12}O_6 \rightarrow 2C_2H_5OH + 2CO_2$$

Ethanol is an excellent solvent and is miscible with water.

Another alcohol, glycerol, is the basic building block of natural fats and oils. The chemical formula for glycerol is $HOCH_2CHOHCH_2OH$ and it has a specific gravity of 1.26 and melts at 18° C, well below our body temperature of 37° C.

Fats and oils

Fats and oils are *glycerides*, that is, esters in which one, two or three fatty acid molecules are attached to a glycerol molecule. Glycerides (also called glycerols) are naturally occurring lipids (fat-soluble components of living cells).

Esters are a class of organic compounds produced by replacing the hydrogen of an acid by a radical such as alkyl or aryl. Many esters occur naturally as oils and fats.

Fats and oils are oily, greasy, or waxy substances, lighter than, and practically insoluble in, water. With the exception of castor oil, they are insoluble in cold alcohol and only sparingly soluble in hot alcohol.

The distinction between fats and oils is that fats are solid at room temperature, whereas oils are liquid, only solidifying at lower temperatures. Waxes are esters of fatty acids with higher alcohols, and are hard solids at ordinary temperatures.

Glycerides are named according to their fatty acid components; for example, tristearin is a *triglyceride* which contains three molecules of stearic acid, whilst oleodistearin contains one molecule of oleic acid and two of stearic acid.

Lard is a triglyceride containing oleic acid, palmitic acid, and stearic acid. Lard can be broken down into substances that have important commercial uses. Olein is an oily substance used as a lubricant, as a burning oil, and in the manufacture of margarine. Palmitin is used to make soap and candles. Stearin is used in the manufacture of soap, ointments, and some kinds of margarine.

Dietary glycerides are typically triglycerides and are sources of stored energy in animals and probably in plant seeds. In mammals they are stored in adipose tissue until needed, at which time they are transported to the liver and broken down to a molecule of glycerol and three molecules of fatty acid. The latter combine with albumin, a protein in blood plasma, and are carried in the bloodstream to sites of utilization.

The types of triglycerides in animals vary with the species and the composition of fats in the food. Many vegetable triglycerides (oils) are liquid at room temperature, unlike those of animals; in addition, they contain a greater variety of fatty acids.

Normally, triglycerides are obtained from foods, but excessive sugar and alcohol consumption can cause them to be synthesized in the body. **High levels of blood triglycerides are associated with increased blood VLDL cholesterol and sugar levels, and are therefore a cause of heart disease.**

Fatty acids contribute from 94 to 96 percent of the total weight of various fats and oils. Because of their preponderant weight in the glyceride molecules and also because they comprise the reactive portion of the molecules, the fatty acids influence greatly both the physical and chemical character of glycerides.

Animal fats are actually a mixture of different glycerides and vary widely in complexity. Some contain only a few component acids, and at the other extreme more than 100 different fatty acids have been identified in butterfat, although many are present in only trace quantities.

Most of the oils and fats are based on about a dozen fatty acids. In considering the composition of a glyceride it is particularly important to distinguish between the saturated acids (acids containing only single bonds between carbon atoms, such as palmitic or stearic), with relatively high melting temperatures, and the unsaturated acids (acids with one or more pairs of carbon atoms joined by double bonds, such as oleic or linoleic), which have lower melting points and are chemically much more reactive.

In addition to triglycerides, foods contain small amounts of phospholipids. These are also esters of fatty acids with glycerol, but contain only two fatty acids per molecule, the third ester to the glycerol being to phosphate and a water-miscible group. They are important constituents of the membranes of all cells. They will emulsify oils in water, and some (for example, lecithin) are commonly used for this purpose as food additives.

Dietary fats and oils

Fats, which provide 9 calories of energy per gram, are the most concentrated of the energy-producing nutrients, so our bodies need only very small amounts. Fats play an important role in building the membranes that surround our cells and in helping blood to clot.

Fat stored in the body cushions vital organs and protects us from extreme cold and heat. Fat is also important for the absorption of the fat-soluble vitamins A, D, E, and K, as well as ß-carotene. Much of the flavour of foods is contained in the fat.

The different fatty acids that make up dietary fats can be classified as saturated or unsaturated.

In *saturated fatty acids* all the carbon atoms carry their full quota of hydrogen atoms, and there are only single bonds between the carbon atoms. Animal fats (eggs, dairy products, and meats) are high in saturated fats and cholesterol, a chemical substance found in all animal fat. Hard animal fats contain relatively more saturated fatty acids than do softer fats and oils from vegetable sources.

Saturated fats raise LDL and VLDL levels and decrease HDL levels and are therefore harmful to the heart and blood vessels. Intake of saturated fats should therefore be limited as much as possible.

In *unsaturated fatty acids* two or more carbon atoms carry only a single hydrogen atom each, and there are one or more double bonds between carbon atoms. Fatty acids with only one double bond are called monounsaturated, those with two or more double bonds are polyunsaturated.

Vegetable fats such as those found in avocados, olives, some nuts, and certain vegetable oils are rich in monounsaturated and polyunsaturated fat.

The temperature at which a fat melts is determined by both the length of the fatty acid chains and also the degree of saturation. Fats containing longer chain fatty acids melt at a higher temperature, while those with more unsaturated fatty acids melt at lower temperatures.

Monounsaturated fats found in olive, canola, and peanut oils appear to decrease LDL and VLDL levels and increase HDL levels.

Polyunsaturated fats found in margarine and sunflower, soybean, corn, and safflower oils are considered more healthful than saturated fats. However, if consumed in excess (more than 10 percent of daily calories), they can decrease the blood levels of HDLs.

Some polyunsaturated fatty acids are dietary essentials in small amounts, since they are the precursors of prostaglandins and other locally acting hormone-like compounds in the body. There are two groups of these compounds, derived from different polyunsaturated fatty acids.

The difference between the two parent fatty acids is the position of the first carbon-carbon double bond counting from the methyl end of the fatty acid. It may be at the 3rd or 6th carbon in, and they are known as the omega-3 and omega-6 fatty acids.

Trans fatty acids result from the partial saturation of oils to harden them to produce margarine and vegetable shortenings.

There is some evidence that high intakes of trans fatty acids are associated with higher incidence of heart disease. It is therefore recommended that intake of trans fatty acids should be limited to 2 per cent of energy intake.

Fat metabolism

In animals the fats in foods are emulsified with digestive secretions containing lipase, an enzyme that hydrolyses at least part of the glycerides. The glycerol, partial glycerol esters, fatty acids, and some glycerides are then absorbed through the intestine and are at least partially recombined to form glycerides and phospholipids. The fat, in the form of microscopic droplets, is transported in the blood to points of use or storage. The fat of an individual animal may vary somewhat according to the composition of fats in the food.

Fats used by or stored in animal tissues come from:

(a) Direct absorption and recombination of dietary fatty acids.

(b) Enzymatic synthesis from carbohydrate intermediates, followed by enzymatic re-synthesis to form the fat characteristic of the animal.

A normal human male has about 15 kg of stored fat, enough to support life for about two months (a woman circa twice this). The breakdown of storage fat during metabolism yields fatty acids, the source of metabolic energy for muscle contraction. The body's adipose tissue is in a constant state of buildup and breakdown, thus ensuring a continual supply of fatty acids.

When reserve fat is mobilized most of it is sent to the liver where fatty acids are partially desaturated by removing hydrogen from the fatty-acid chains to produce unsaturated or double bonds between carbon atoms. This facilitates subsequent oxidation in other tissues. Fatty acids may also be oxidized directly in the various tissues as well as in the liver.

Fatty-acid metabolism occurs by oxidation in successive two- and four-carbon stages. Intermediate products could be acetoacetate and acetate groups. If the mechanism is faulty, acetone is formed and excreted (acetonuria). The final products of normal metabolism are carbon dioxide and water.

Carbohydrates and proteins

These include sugars, starches and cellulose. They are produced in plants by photosynthesis. Common sugar or sucrose has the formula $C_{12}H_{22}O_{11}$ and is the most heavily produced organic substance.

Carbohydrates form the bulk of the human diet and the digestive process breaks them all down into '6-carbon' sugars which are carried to the liver and converted to glycogen, an amorphous, tasteless, starch-like polysaccharide compound $(C_6H_{10}O_5)n$.

This is stored in the liver or the muscles and converted as required to glucose, the formula for which is $C_6H_{12}O_6$, and it is this which is 'blood sugar', the body's major source of energy.

One of the end products of glucose metabolism in the muscles is lactic acid and this is carried back to the liver and some of it converted back to glycogen.

Blood sugar levels rise soon after a large meal but increased insulin production keeps blood sugar from rising excessively as the carbohydrates are broken down into their constituent sugar molecules.

Proteins are made up of amino acids and are broken into these by the digestive system. Dietary amino acids from ingested protein are circulated to the liver, where they are either cycled into the production of specific human proteins, or converted to glucose by removing the amino group (deamination), a process called gluconeogenesis in which ammonia is released from amino acids and converted into urea.

The glycogen and glucose from excessive carbohydrate (especially sugar and alcohol) and protein intake undergo enzymatic resynthesis into triglycerides which are stored as body fat.

Cholesterol

Cholesterol is a waxy sterol, a type of alcohol that is part of the steroid group of compounds. It is present in the blood plasma and in all animal tissues, particularly the brain. Its molecular formula is $C_{27}H_{46}O$ and in its pure state it is a white, crystalline substance that is odourless and tasteless.

Cholesterol is a primary component of the membrane that surrounds each cell and it is the starting material or an intermediate compound from which the body synthesizes bile acids, steroid and sex hormones, and vitamin D.

Cholesterol circulates in the bloodstream and is synthesized by the liver and several other organs, and is therefore a nonessential nutrient that does not need to be obtained from food.

Human beings also ingest considerable amounts of cholesterol in the course of a normal diet. A compensatory system regulates the amount of cholesterol synthesized by the liver, with the increased dietary intake of cholesterol resulting in decreased synthesis of the compound in the liver.

When saturated solid fats are added to the diet, the amount of cholesterol in the blood increases, but when liquid, unsaturated fats or oils (particularly the polyunsaturated type) replace solid fat, the amount of cholesterol decreases.

Foods high in unsaturated fats include olive oil and oily fish.

Cholesterol and its derivatives are secreted through the oil glands of the skin to act as a lubricant and protective covering for the hair and skin. Lanolin, a grease extracted from raw sheep wool and composed largely of cholesterol esters, has a variety of commercial uses in lubricants, leather preservatives, ointments, and cosmetics.

Lipoproteins and cholesterol transport

Lipoproteins are substances containing both lipid (fat) and protein. They occur in both soluble complexes, as in egg yolk and mammalian blood plasma, and insoluble ones, as in cell membranes.

Cholesterol is insoluble in water so it must be bound to the large molecules of lipoproteins to be transported through the bloodstream and lymphatic fluid.

Three types of lipoprotein are involved in this function:

(a) Low-density lipoproteins (LDLs) and very-low-density lipoproteins (VLDL). These transport cholesterol from its site of synthesis in the liver to the body's cells where it is used for various purposes.

About 70 percent of all cholesterol in the blood is carried by LDL particles and LDL-bound cholesterol is primarily responsible for the atherosclerotic buildup of plaque-forming cholesterol deposits on the blood vessel walls.

(b) High-density lipoproteins (HDLs) transport excess or unused cholesterol from the body's tissues back to the liver where it is broken down to bile acids and then excreted.

HDL particles may actually reduce or retard atherosclerotic buildups and are thus beneficial to health.

Body cells extract cholesterol from the blood by means of tiny coated pits (receptors) on their surfaces; these receptors bind with the LDL particles (and their attached cholesterol) and draw them from the blood into the cell. There are limits to how much cholesterol a body cell can take in, however, so that diets high in cholesterol and thence saturated fats result in cholesterol accumulating in the interior walls of blood vessels.

An inherited genetic disorder called *familial hypercholesterolemia* reduces LDL-receptor formation, resulting in high blood cholesterol levels. Other factors that increase cholesterol levels include thyroid gland malfunction, kidney disease, diabetes, and the use of various medicines, including certain diuretics.

Several hereditary genetic disorders, called *hyper-lipoproteinemias,* involve excessive concentrations of lipoproteins in the blood. Conversely, diseases called hypolipoproteinemias involve abnormally reduced lipoprotein levels in the blood.

Atherosclerosis

The word atherosclerosis is derived from the two Greek words atheroma, meaning *porridge*, and scleros, meaning *hard,* an observation that might serve quite well to describe nature of atherosclerosis.

This disease affects the innermost of the three layers of the artery. This layer is lined with a dense, single-celled surface that in a healthy person prevents any abnormal substances in the blood from entering the thickness of the wall. It also prevents clotting of the blood.

It has repeatedly been shown experimentally that diets high in saturated fats result in high blood cholesterol levels and thence deposits of cholesterol and other fatty substances on this inner layer.

If such diets are continued, these fatty streaks thicken, immune response causing invasion by white blood cells. If lipid deposition continues the WBCs become engorged and die, forming *foam cells,* resulting in plaques with a core of cholesterol, other fats, and degenerate muscle cells and other debris. Plaques then develop a few blood vessels and a dense fibrous cap of calcified connective tissue, these stubborn cyst-like lesions being called fibrolipid plaques.

The main effect of arterial plaques is that by growing out towards the centre of the vessel, they impede the flow of blood to an organ.

The blood carries the fibrous protein clotting factor *fibrinogen* which causes blood clotting. Because plaques no longer have the properties of healthy vessel lining, the fibrinogen in the blood can readily form *thrombi* on their surface. These may then detach, producing *embolisms* that migrate to and block smaller blood vessels in the heart or brain.

Reduced blood flow as a result of coronary atherosclerosis is the cause of attacks of *angina pectoris* during exertion.

Atherosclerosis can all too easily close off the moderately sized coronary arteries, resulting in *coronary thrombosis* or heart attack which is still fatal in 50% of cases, often within hours.

Atherosclerosis often clogs the four arteries in the neck, resulting in *cerebral thrombosis* and sudden shutdown in blood supply to the brain, often resulting in brain damage. Atherosclerosis also weakens blood vessels, leading to haemorrhagic strokes which are often fatal.

It also causes *peripheral artery disease* (PAD) which can completely block blood vessels in the legs. This results in *stasis dermatitis, stasis ulcers,* and in extreme cases *gangrene* which often results in amputation. PAD may also release clots that cause heart attacks (Donatelle, 2011).

Causes of atherosclerosis

There is no doubt that atherosclerosis is caused by elevated blood lipid levels (for example, cholesterol > 240 mg/dl) which may be the result of dietary excesses (especially saturated fats) and be exacerbated by smoking.

The disease usually starts in childhood and develops slowly. Its effects rarely become apparent before the age of 40 or 50 when heart attacks are common in men mainly because women have higher HDL levels so long as they are secreting the female hormone oestrogen. After the menopause, however, atherosclerosis tends to progress more rapidly in women. Strokes occur later and affect the sexes about equally.

Hypercholesterolemia and hyperlipoproteinemias greatly increase cholesterol levels and thence the progression of atherosclerosis.

Plasma cholesterol is also raised secondary to certain diseases, for example, hypothyroidism, some types of kidney disease, bile duct obstruction, and diabetes mellitus.

Insulin resistance, smoking and other factors can raise blood levels of ADMA (asymmetric dimethylarginine), a situation associated with higher triglyceride and homocysteine levels. ADMA blocks nitric oxide (NO, the endothelial-derived relaxation factor or EDRF) production and is believed to be a mechanism by which all risk factors adversely affect the endothelium (Cooke & Zimmer, 2002).

The importance of oxidation

A major factor in the development of atherosclerosis is oxidation of cholesterol within the arteries. To understand the situation a useful example of a comparable oxidation process is that of oxidation of glucose by Fehling's solution, which is copper hydroxide dissolved in an alkaline solution of sodium nitrate:

$$CH_2OH(COH_2)_4\ COH + 2Cu(OH)_2$$
$$\rightarrow CH_2OH(COH_2)_4\ COOH + Cu_2O(precipitated) + 2H_2O$$

Here precipitation of red cuprous oxide is used as a diagnostic test for glucose but our interest here is that the aldehyde group COH at the end of the glucose molecule is oxidized to form a COOH carboxyl group. These are characteristic of the carboxylic acids which are the building blocks for fats (Medeiros, 1971).

Thus this reaction is an example of how unused sugars in our diet are converted to fat and stored for later use.

It is when such oxidation of cholesterol in the blood occurs to excess that the process of atherosclerosis begins, resulting in fatty streaks some of which eventually develop into plaques filled with dead cells and other debris and covered by fibrous scar tissue. Containing material like pus these are like an abscess and are prone to rupture, 'throwing' clots which often cause heart attacks and strokes.

When cholesterol is put to its proper use, however, it is transported to various sites for a variety of uses, including to form cell membranes, artery linings, and coatings for nerves and the body's organs.

For these applications, a process loosely comparable to the polymerization process used to manufacture polyethylene from ethylene occurs to form a continuous material.

Combating atherosclerosis

Plasma cholesterol (total and LDL) can be consistently reduced by changing intake of fats and oils as follows:

(1) Reduce total fat intake (preferably to 10 - 15% of calories).

(2) Reduce saturated fat and cholesterol intake as much as possible.

(3) Reduce energy intake if overweight.

(4) Increase intake of vegetables, fruits, and whole grain cereals.

(5) Moderately increase intake of polyunsaturated and some monounsaturated oils, especially EPA and DHA.

Exercise, dietary supplements and other measures are also important and these are discussed in other chapters.

Note that, whilst total cholesterol and LDL-C levels should be kept as low as possible, it is desirable to increase HDL-C levels and sound diet and exercise will help achieve this.

Finally, note that *oxycholesterol* found in fried and processed food, and especially in fast food, is a particularly damaging form of dietary cholesterol which should be avoided as far as possible.

11. Fats and Cholesterol

Chapter 12

TACKLING CHOLESTEROL
AND HOMOCYSTEINE

> *If cholesterol is petty crime, then homocysteine is grand larceny.*
> *Elevated homocysteine levels triple the risk*
> *of heart attacks and stroke.*
> *Real Age, Are You as Young as You Can Be?*
> Michael Roizen (2001).

Introduction

Early in Chapter One a number of early theories about the causes of atherosclerosis were outlined. Now it is clear beyond dispute that unsatisfactory blood lipid levels are the primary cause of atherosclerosis, the most common problems being excessive total cholesterol, *low-density lipoprotein* (LDL) and *triglyceride* levels and also *high-density lipoprotein* (HDL) levels that are too low.

Levels of *homocysteine*, an amino acid that can build up in excess in the blood, are also thought to be a major factor in arterial damage and an introductory discussion of how to tackle the problems of high cholesterol and homocysteine levels is given in this chapter.

The effects of cholesterol

The body manufactures much of its cholesterol requirements so dietary cholesterol intake should be limited. High intake of saturated fats, refined carbohydrates and sugars, however, also raise blood cholesterol levels and lead to arterial cholesterol deposits.

In fact, cholesterol deposits begin to build up in our childhood when sugar may become our first addiction and cakes, biscuits, chocolate, fatty snack foods and the like begin to clog our cardiovascular system.

Thus by middle age some people have arterial obstruction caused by cholesterol plaques and this may be in all of the blood vessels connected to the heart and involve obstructions of up to 90% and complete blockage of some 'secondary' blood vessels.

These atherosclerotic plaques deprive the underlying tissue of oxygen. The result is arteriosclerosis when cell death occurs in the anoxic tissue and it hardens, becoming less elastic. This tissue is then more vulnerable to some sudden stress peak so that ultimately aneurysm may result.

Thus cholesterol may lead to congestive heart failure or stroke, and also to catastrophic haemorrhage of a small vessel in the brain.

First, however, cholesterol will clog small capillaries throughout our body and this will increase our blood pressure, perhaps leading to permanent prescription of medication to control it.

In addition, cholesterol clogs arteries in the heart and gradually reduces its efficiency. Eventually the weakened heart muscle may fibrillate, going into a torsional non-pumping mode, at which point we have only a minute or two to live.

Should we live long enough and avoid all the disasters just described clogged capillaries in our brain will give us senile dementia of the Alzheimer type (SDAT).

In other words, as the equations given in Chapter 25 for heart risk as a function of cholesterol levels demonstrate, cholesterol is a matter that deserves serious consideration from as early as possible in our lives, particularly because arteries damaged by atherosclerosis gradually become 'stickier' so that atherosclerotic plaques accumulate at an exponential rate (Rath, 2001b).

Study finds in favour of niacin

A study of 8341 men, aged from 30 to 64, who had suffered a myocardial infarction at least three months before entering the study, extended from 1966 to 1975. It tested five drugs for lowering cholesterol against placebo. At the end of the 9-year study 6000 men remained alive but only niacin had decreased the death rate significantly from all causes, reducing mortality by 11% and increasing longevity by 2 years. The death rate from cancer was also decreased (Canner et al., 1986).

Kowalski's "8 Week Cholesterol Cure"

Robert Kowalski had had two quadruple bypasses and one heart attack and was swimming a mile of laps in a pool from three to five times a week. Nevertheless, his concerned doctor found that his blood cholesterol levels were still too high (Kowalski, 1987).

Kowalski stumbled across an article in the *Journal of the American Medical Association* saying: "*Nicotinic acid in doses of three to twelve 500 mg tablets daily will also lower the plasma LDL level 15% to 30%, and it is also effective in the reduction of VLDL levels. It also increases HDL levels.*"

Here nicotinic acid or niacin is a form of vitamin B3, LDL is the 'bad' cholesterol which can readily form clots and plaques, and HDL is the stable 'good' cholesterol needed to carry excess cholesterol back to the liver from the arteries. VLDL is very low density lipoprotein which is even more dangerous to the arteries than LDL.

Kowalski then found that taking a gram of niacin three times a day for just eight weeks, along with a diet low in fat and high in fibre (particularly oat bran), reduced his total cholesterol level by 40%, whereas previously a highly restrictive diet had only reduced it by 5.5%. His ratio of total cholesterol to HDL was an acceptable 3.4.

Table 12.1. Results of Kowalski's 8-week cholesterol reduction program.

	Participant compliance	
	Good	Low
Total cholesterol reduction %	31.7	22.1
LDL decrease %	47.5	32.6
HDL increase %	60.6	43.9
Triglycerides decrease %	42.1	41.2

His 8-week program was then tried on 20 people at a hospital cardiac rehabilitation centre, two of these being doctors, and the results are summarized in Table 12.1. The fifteen people who stuck to the program obtained reductions in total cholesterol of from 30 to 50%, HDL levels doubled in some cases, and levels of triglycerides, another type of blood fat, were cut by almost half.

McGowan's case studies

Mary McGowan, one of the leading experts on cholesterol in the USA, also found high dosage niacin successful as a means of improving cholesterol levels. McGowan's recommended dosage is 750 mg daily for two weeks and then 1500 mg daily for six weeks followed by reevaluation of cholesterol levels (McGowan, 1998), after which dosage may be increased to 2000 - 3000 mg daily according to the test results.

Her book tells of nine case studies in which people had experienced the pains of thromboses and heart attacks and been found to have high cholesterol levels

Some of these people had a history of high cholesterol levels dating back to their twenties, two of them having suffered familial combined hyperlipidemia (FCH). FCH is an inherited genetic disorder that causes abnormally high cholesterol levels, sometimes resulting in heart attacks as early as at 20 years of age.

Most of these people had had coronary arteries obstructed by as much as 90%, requiring surgery ranging from angioplasty to clear them, to coronary bypass operations.

Then they sought to reduce their cholesterol levels by a combination of exercise, careful diets with minimum fat, and prescription drugs or niacin.

One case study was a man with severe arterial obstruction at the age of 38. He was a little too young for bypass surgery the grafts of which last only from 1 to 15 years and the obstructions were not more than 70% so he was told to give up smoking, go on a low fat diet, and given an exercise and cardiac medication program.

Nearly four years later he had severe pains in his left arm and dizziness and nausea. Tests now showed severe artery obstruction and heart deterioration and a bypass operation was carried out.

After the operation his cholesterol levels (in mg per decilitre) were those shown in Table 12.2.

These were poor results considering he had already been on a diet, exercise and medication program for years.

He was told to very carefully eliminate fat from his diet as far as possible, make his exercise more vigourous by aiming for a target heart rate, and to take niacin.

Table 12.2. Cholesterol results for bypass operation patient.

Total cholesterol	251 mg/dl	Desirable < 200
LDL cholesterol	172 mg/dl	Desirable < 100
HDL cholesterol	41 mg/dl	Desirable > 45
		Desirable Total/HDL < 4
Triglycerides	191 mg/dl	Desirable < 150
Lipoprotein (a)	95 mg/dl	Desirable < 20

After 6 and 14 weeks the test results were those shown in Table 12.3. The results after just 6 weeks were almost acceptable.

Table 12.3. Improved cholesterol levels for bypass operation patient.

	6 weeks	14 weeks	Desirable
Total cholesterol	166	155 < 200	
LDL cholesterol	89	84	<100
HDL cholesterol	43	48	>45
Triglycerides	168	116	<150
Lipoprotein(a)		32	<20

After 14 weeks his cholesterol levels were acceptable except for the level of lipoprotein(a), another blood lipid similar to LDL which is, according to some experts, genetically predetermined and can only be brought down with the use of medication. After two years, however, the patient's lipoprotein(a) level had been reduced to just 16, demonstrating that niacin is effective in reducing lipoprotein(a) levels.[1]

That Kowalski's plan and McGowan's case study produced good results after only 6 - 8 weeks is strongly indicative of the effectiveness of niacin in reducing cholesterol and triglyceride levels.

McGowan (1998) recommends LDL < 100 to regress atheroma but analysis of the results of four recent intensive statins therapy trials of 1455 patients found that it was reduction of LDL to < 87.5 and increase of HDL to > 45 which resulted in regression (Nicholls et al., 2007).

---

[1] As noted in Chapter 2, Lp(a) levels can also be reduced by taking lysine and vitamin C.

Side-effects of niacin

Many people experience 'hot flush' feelings in the face and perhaps upper body with high doses of niacin. As little as 100 mg can cause a slight effect but 500 - 1000 mg may cause some people discomfort. Long-term dosages of 2 grams or more daily can cause liver problems.

The flushing symptoms can be overcome by using slow-release niacin formulations (Kowalski, 2006) but there is a greater risk of liver damage with prolonged use of these (Cooper, 1996).

The alternative form of vitamin B3 is nicotinamide, a metabolite of niacin, and this is far less potent and does not cause flushing symptoms. It improves energy metabolism but does not affect cholesterol levels much.

Triglycerides

Very low density lipoprotein is primarily made up of triglycerides and a rough estimate of VLDL level is obtained by dividing the triglyceride level by 5.[2] Then total cholesterol level is approximately given by

$$TC = HDL + LDL + VLDL = HDL + LDL + TG/5$$

and the measured levels in Tables 12.2 and 12.3 fit this equation reasonably well.

High triglyceride levels tend to be a marker for low HDL levels and small dense LDL, a more dangerous form of LDL.

To reduce triglyceride levels reduce simple sugars and refined sugars in one's diet, for example sugar, syrups, ice cream, confectionery (especially chocolate with fat as well), fruit, jams, cakes and pastry.

Fat and alcohol (which increase trigycleride levels substantially) should also be minimized.

Total calories should also be reduced to lose excess body fat and exercise should be sufficient to burn up a substantial number of calories.

Exercise reduces triglyceride levels rapidly and also increases HDL levels.

---

[2] VLDL is a precursor to LDL because VLDL particles carry both triglycerides and cholesterol, becoming LDL when they 'drop off' their triglyceride component (Westcott, 2002).

Homocysteine

There is a strong link between homocysteine and vascular disease: "More than 42% of people with cerebrovascular disease, 30% of those with cardiovascular disease, and 28% of those with peripheral vascular disease have homocysteine levels that are too high" (Roizen, 2001).

Homocysteine is synthesized in the body from methionine, an amino acid made by digestion of proteins, and is carried in the bloodstream by albumin and haemoglobin. Methionine is also found in animal protein so that diets high in this raise homocysteine levels.

Homocysteine interferes with synthesis of collagen and elastin required for healthy arteries. It also irritates arterial linings, causing small lesions which initiate plaques. It may also oxidize LDL, further growing plaques.

Before menopause women's homocysteine levels are about 10 to 15% less than men's, one of the reasons why women are less prone to heart disease pre-menopause (another is that pre-menopausal women have 15 - 20% higher HDL levels).

Taking 400 mcg of folate a day, an amount difficult to obtain and absorb from food alone, plus vitamins B6 and B12, can reduce homocysteine levels to acceptable levels in three months.

Recent trials have found that lowering homocysteine levels with B vitamins does reduce incidence of heart attacks and strokes but not death rates from well-established disease ('Homocysteine', Wikipedia, 2008), suggesting that, whilst lowering homocysteine levels with B vitamins will help prevent atherosclerosis, supplements such as those discussed in the next two chapters are needed to *reverse* it.

Circulating homocysteine is also biomarker for the likelihood of microalbuminuria (MA) of thence chronic kidney disease (CKD).

In addition, homocysteine is also a marker for brain shrinkage, and thus a forerunner of dementia, heart disease and eventual death. For this reason, along with the length of the telomeres found on the end the chromosomes in each cell, homocysteine levels may be useful as a predictor of likely longevity.

Lipoprotein (a)

Whilst there is a strong correlation between cholesterol levels and heart disease, lipoprotein (a), a type of LDL, is now thought to be the main cause of atherosclerotic plaques (see Chapter 2).

Rath (2001b) reports that niacin in doses of 2 - 4 gm daily can lower Lp(a) levels by up to 36%, but comparison of Tables 12.2 and 12.3 shows a much better reduction in Lp(a) with high dosages of niacin.

Alternatively, smaller amounts of niacin, along with the ingredients of the Pauling Therapy (see Chapter 2), namely vitamin C and amino acids lysine and proline, may reduce Lp(a) levels and even regress plaque deposits in arteries (Rath, 2001b).

Conclusions

[1] The health of the endothelium, the lining of the blood vessels, is closely related to and just as important as blood cholesterol levels (Cooke and Zimmer, 2002).

[2] Cholesterol and other lipid levels can be reduced by avoiding fat and excess sugar in the diet, and exercising to remove excess body fat.

Plenty of fibre in the diet also helps reduce fat absorption from food.

Omega-3 fish oils, soy protein, phytosterols found in kidney beans and other vegetables, and garlic in the diet also help reduce cholesterol levels. Fish oil and garlic oil capsules can also be used as supplements.

[3] Niacin is the most effective agent for raising HDL levels, resulting in increases of up to 35%. Niacin also lowers LDL, VLDL, triglyceride, lipoprotein (a) and small LDL levels. Several clinical trials have found niacin effective, alone or in combination with other drugs, in slowing or even regressing atherosclerosis, and preventing coronary events (Expert panel, 2001; Linus Pauling Institute, Oregon, 2009).

[4] Prescription drugs, some incorporating niacin, are available for reducing cholesterol levels. Some of these are very expensive and, like niacin, involve a risk of liver toxicity so that regular liver function tests should be done. The most effective of the cholesterol lowering drugs are the statins which lower cholesterol levels as much as 30 to 40% (Cooke and Zimmer, 2002). Research by the British Medical Council and the Medical Research Council of Australia found that statins reduce risk of heart attack and stroke by about a third (*The Australian,* Sept. 28, 2005).

12. Tackling Cholesterol and Homocysteine

Until recently statins were relatively ineffective at raising HDL levels and niacin was *"somewhat better in this regard"* (Cooke and Zimmer, 2002). As a result nearly all the human and animal trials which found evidence of atherosclerosis regression included niacin as part of an aggressive combination agent strategy (Blankenhorn & Dodis, 1993).

The latest statins, however, do increase HDL (Nissen et al., 2006).

[5} An alternative that is available over the shelf is Policosanol which contains sugar cane wax alcohols and has been claimed clinically proven to be effective in reducing LDL levels and increasing HDL levels. Reports and trials of the effectiveness of Policosonal are discussed in Chapter 13.

[6] Antioxidant supplementation also helps reduce cholesterol levels, especially in conjunction with an appropriate diet and exercise program.

In the 1970s Dr Emil Ginter found that less than 1 gram of vitamin C daily lowered cholesterol by about 10% in 7 weeks, and that dosage of 1 gram reduced triglyceride levels by almost 50% (Murray, 1977).

Another finding was that 50 to 90 mg of oral vitamin E daily for 1 to 5 weeks reduced cholesterol levels by 32 mg%, "with the maximal effect within eight days," whilst 100,000 IU vitamin A and 60 mg vitamin E intramuscularly for 7 to 20 days reduced cholesterol levels by 70 mg% (Cheraskin et al., 1975).

[7] Exercise lowers LDL levels and increases HDL levels (Cooke and Zimmer, 2002). Even a daily glass of wine helps increase HDL levels, but not if exercise has already achieved this. Stress, however, is bad for cholesterol levels and cardiovascular health in general.

[8] A recent study in the British Medical Journal concluded that the amino acid homocysteine in the blood is a cause of cardiovascular disease. Homocysteine tends to build up in the body over the years and may be as harmful, if not more so, than cholesterol, and McGowan's hospital Cholesterol Management Centre was introducing tests for its level at the time of publication of her excellent book (1998).

She concluded that less than 10 micromoles per litre was an acceptable homocysteine level, while Wescott (2002) suggests 12 mmol/l or less.

The acceptable amount of total cholesterol is about 5 mmol/l, not greatly dissimilar, emphasizing the importance of controlling both cholesterol and homocysteine levels.

Homocysteine levels can be reduced by taking folate and ensuring adequate intake of vitamins B6 and B12. Most diets should have adequate B6 and tablets containing 500 mg of folate, some with 500 mcg of B12, are available in supermarkets. Taken daily these tablets will normalize homocysteine levels in three months.

[9] Some studies have found that niacin may increase homocysteine levels, a motivation to limit dosage and use niacin in combination with other agents which alter lipid levels by different mechanisms.

(10) Cholesterol levels should be kept about 30 mg/dl lower during pregnancy to reduce the risk of such problems as gestational diabetes (Masharani, 2008).

Other natural supplements that may help improve cholesterol levels and prevent, or even reverse, vascular and heart disease are discussed in the following chapter.

Chapter 13

DIETARY SUPPLEMENTS FOR CARDIOVASCULAR DISEASE

*It has been demonstrated that niacin therapy reduces
the risk of a second heart attack and can reduce the rate
of coronary heart disease build-up in the coronary arteries
as well as actually regressing it in some cases.*
Before The Heart Attacks
Robert Superko, with Laura Tucker (2004).

Introduction

Many natural supplements have been claimed to be able to improve blood cholesterol levels and thus help prevent, or even reverse heart disease and vascular disease in general. One of these, niacin, was discussed at some length in the preceding chapter and another, Policosanol, briefly mentioned. The present chapter discusses several other natural supplements which may help in tackling heart disease.

Prostaglandins

Two of the supplements discussed in this chapter stimulate biosynthesis of the *prostaglandin* PGI_2. Prostaglandins are one of three types of *eicosanoid* and are found in all mammalian organs. The others are the related *thromboxanes*, which are found in blood platelets, and the *leukotrienes*, whose biological effects include respiratory, vascular, and intestinal activities.

Prostaglandins are hormone-like substances of which at least 16 have been isolated. They are powerful *vasodilators* that relax the muscles in the walls of blood vessels so that their diameters become larger and there is less resistance to blood flow. Thromboxanes, on the other hand, are powerful *vasoconstrictors* in the same setting.

Discovered by Sir John Vane and his UK research team in the early 1970s, the important prostaglandin *prostacyclin* or PGI_2 is synthesized in the walls of blood vessels and inhibits aggregation of platelets to form blood clots.

Conversely, thromboxanes strongly stimulate clot formation. Thromboxanes are synthesized within the platelets themselves and are released. The platelets adhere to one another and to blood vessel walls.

Through prostaglandin and thromboxane mechanisms, clotting is prevented when it is unnecessary and takes place when it is necessary.

Platelets adhere in arteries that are affected by the process of atherosclerosis, forming plaques along the interior surface of the vessel wall. This type of platelet aggregation and clotting leads to blocking (occlusion) of the vessel, the most common cause of heart attack (coronary artery occlusion).

The enzyme cyclooxygenase plays a role in biosynthesis of thromboxanes. This enzyme is inhibited by *aspirin*, the reason for the widespread recommendation that those at risk of a coronary occlusion take aspirin daily.

Thromboxanes, along with *endothelin*, a protein produced by the endothelium, also cause arteries to spasm and eventually thicken.

Prostaglandins also play a pivotal role in the immune response of histamine-induced local dilation of capillaries that results in increased blood flow and *inflammation* of the affected area. The capillaries become more permeable, leading to the escape of infection-fighting fluid and white blood cells from the blood into the surrounding tissues. These changes are mediated by prostaglandins and leukotrienes. Thus, effective treatment to suppress inflammation in inflammatory but noninfectious diseases, such as rheumatoid arthritis, is to treat the patient with inhibitors of prostaglandin synthesis, such as aspirin.

Prostaglandins also play important roles in the digestive process and in endocrine function.

Niacin

Niacin or nicotinic acid is a form of vitamin B3. It is widely used in the USA, often in conjunction with prescription medications, particularly statins. Kowalski (1987) showed that taking 3 grams daily reduced blood cholesterol levels by up to 40% in just 8 weeks (see Table 12.1).

He obtained even better results with 1.5 grams daily of a slow-release niacin formulation (Kowalski, 2006).

Note that long-term high dosage (more than about a gram daily) of niacin may risk liver damage, slow-release niacin formulations increasing this risk (Cooper, 1996), so that as a precaution blood tests should be made for liver enzymes as well as for cholesterol and triglyceride levels.

For longer term niacin supplementation Lierberman and Bruning (1997) recommend 250 - 500 mg, and Cooke and Zimmer (2002) recommend 300 - 600 mg with higher dosages only if cholesterol levels remain unsatisfactory.

Niacin has the following effects:

(1) It inhibits a key enzyme for hepatic triglyceride (TG) synthesis, resulting in accelerated intracellular hepatic apoprotein B degradation and decreased secretion (and levels) of VLDL and LDL. It may also lower TG levels by decreasing fatty acid mobilization from adipose tissues.

It also increases HDL half-life (and levels), and thus reverse cholesterol transport, by inhibiting action of hepatic HDL receptors and thus retarding hepatic catabolism of HDL-apoA1 (Kamanna & Kashyap, 2008).

Niacin also reduces lipoprotein (a) levels, whereas most statins do not reduce Lp(a) or increase HDL. It may also increase the activity of lipoprotein lipase (LPL) which lowers triglycerides and increases HDL, whilst inhibiting production of dangerous small LDL by decreasing the activity of hepatic lipase (Superko, 2004).

(2) It stimulates the production of the prostaglandin PGI_2 (Kowalski, 1987; Heber, 1998) and thence has the following effects:
(a) Blood vessels are relaxed, thereby increasing flow and reducing blood pressure.
(b) Platelet clumping and thus formation of blood clots is reduced.
(c) Sticking of white blood cells to the walls of blood vessels is prevented.
(d) Reduction of oxidative stress and inflammation of blood vessels.
(e) Thickening and hardening of blood vessels is reduced so that they remain more flexible.

(3) Taken for the long term (several months up to a year or more) atherosclerotic plaques may be reduced.

In doses well above its RDI of around 20 mg niacin is renowned for the flushing effect it causes in the upper body. This is the inflammatory effect of prostaglandins described in the previous section. Except in the most extreme cases this is not a cause for concern and flushing symptoms can be reduced by taking a small amount of aspirin before taking niacin.

The effectiveness of niacin in lowering cholesterol levels is exemplified in Tables 12.1 and 12.3. The nicotinamide form of vitamin B3, on the other hand, has little or no effect upon cholesterol levels.

One current website claims that 120 mg potassium iodide and 15 mg of niacin daily can reverse atherosclerotic clogging of the arteries. This is too good to be true as even most multivitamin and mineral tablets provide approximately these amounts of these nutrients.

Potassium iodide was, in fact, found to reduce cholesterol levels and prevent atherosclerotic lesions in 11 of 12 rabbits fed cholesterol for a few months (Turner, 1933). Further work found that this was only a short-term effect for about 4 months (Turner and Bidwell, 1935), other control-group-based work with rabbits and rats finding no reduction in cholesterol levels or atherosclerosis at all (Friedman et al., 1956).

EPA and DHA

EPA (eicosapentaenoic acid) and DHA (docosahexaenoic acid) are two important omega-3 fatty acids found in fish oils.[1] Fish oil capsules rich in EPA and DHA can reduce cholesterol and related problems because, like niacin, they stimulate synthesis of a form of PGI_2, resulting in the following effects:

(1) They reduce triglyceride levels and increase HDL levels.

(2) and (3) as for niacin in the preceding section.

(4) Through the action of superoxide dismutase (SOD) they help the body dispose of harmful free radicals.

For therapeutic purposes 3 or 4 grams per day is recommended (Carper, 2002) but for long-term general health purposes a single 1000 mg capsule daily is sufficient (Cooke and Zimmer, 2002).

Fish oils tend to increase LDL slightly. To prevent this garlic powder can be taken, in one study the result with 900 mg of garlic powder daily being 34% less triglycerides and 10% less LDL (Carper, 2002).

Intake of omega-3 fatty acids can also reduce risk of cardiac arrhythmias and thence heart attack within a month, whereas cholesterol reduction takes 2 to 3 years to reap the same benefit (Carper, 2002).

Fish oils may help shrink plaques by replacing bad fats in artery walls with 'good fats' (Carper, 2000). They also reduce platelet stickiness, thus helping break up blood clots, and some polyunsaturated plant seed oils also reduce platelet stickiness.

---

[1] The liver converts only 5% of plant omega-3 (ALA, see Glossary) to EPA.

In one study taking 6 grams of fish oil for 3 months, then 3 grams for 21 months, resulted in significant reduction of atherosclerotic plaques and cardiovascular events (von Schacky et al., 1999).

Garlic

Garlic has antiplatelet activity which may be owing to stimulation of NO production (see the next section re NO) and also reduces BP slightly (Cooke and Zimmer, 2002). Because it contains compounds such as allicin, S-allylcysteine, ajoene and diallyl disulphide, most studies find that garlic lowers cholesterol levels by 7 to 15% (Carper, 2000).

In one study of 432 heart attack patients, eating 2 or 3 fresh garlic cloves daily reduced fatalities after two years by half, and by two-thirds after three years (Carper, 2000).

A 4-year randomized, double-blind, placebo-controlled German study of 280 adults recently published in *Atherosclerosis* found that those taking 900 mg of garlic daily had up to 82% less arterial plaque volume than the placebo group, suggesting that garlic may indeed regress atherosclerosis, or *"clear the arteries,"* as Dioscorides suggested in the first century AD.

L-arginine

A non-essential (i.e., it is synthesized in the body) amino acid[2] which increases production of the *endothelial-derived relaxation factor* (EDRF) nitric oxide (NO) which is carried by hemoglobin and relaxes blood vessel walls, thereby helping control local blood pressure.

Conversely, the amino acid ADMA (asymmetric dimethylarginine) blocks production of NO. ADMA levels increase in the blood after a high-fat or high-carbohydrate meal and are associated with raised triglyceride, cholesterol and homocysteine levels and also insulin resistance. Indeed, Cooke and Zimmer (2002) found ADMA levels to be "a better indicator of endothelial health than cholesterol."

ADMA can be removed by excretion or broken down by DDAH (dimethyl-arginine dimethylaminohydrolase). DDAH is very sensitive to oxidative stress and can be strengthened by taking antioxidants.

---

[2] Arginine plays a role in protein breakdown to produce urea, the principal form in which mammals excrete nitrogen. It is essential for infants.

Cooke found that intravenous dosage of L-arginine gave immediate improvement in blood vessel function and to treat heart disease he advocates that 3 - 9 grams of L-arginine be taken daily as a dietary supplement (Cooke & Zimmer, 2002). This will result in:

(1) Increased NO production.

(2) and (3) as in the preceding section on niacin.

(4) Reduction in free radicals.

Increased NO not only prevents arterial white blood cell absorption, it also shrinks plaques by killing WBCs in them (Cooke and Zimmer, 2002).

Higher range doses may be used to treat serious symptoms and Cooke obtained excellent results in treating debilitating peripheral vascular disease and angina with L-arginine in as little as two weeks.

L-arginine can also help reduce impotence in men (Kowalski, 2006).

The average Western diet contains from 1 - 4 gm of L-arginine so that for general health relatively little or no supplementation may be needed. Note also that antioxidants such as vitamins C and E, and selenium, help preserve NO (Cooke and Zimmer, 2002).

Policosanal

Policosanal is a blend of sugar cane wax alcohols which is claimed to reduce cholesterol levels in 85% of people within 8 weeks.

Policosanol reduces the activity of an enzyme involved in conversion of acetylCoA to cholesterol and also increases clearance of LDL cholesterol by increasing the number of cellular receptors in HDL.

In randomized studies involving over 1,500 people Policosanal has been found to reduce LDL cholesterol by over 20%.

These results largely stem from a single lab in Cuba, however, and further confirmatory studies are needed (Cooke and Zimmer, 2002).

Indeed, a German study carried out from September 2000 to May 2001 and published in JAMA, found Policosanol ineffective (News-Medical.Net, 2006). The multicentre, randomized, double-blind, placebo-controlled trial was on 143 patients with high cholesterol or blood fats or lipids and having either:

(a) Baseline LDL-C levels of at least 150 mg/dL and either no or one cardiovascular risk factor other than known coronary heart disease,

(b) LDL-C levels of between 150 and 189 mg/dL and 2 or more risk factors.

The patients were randomized into 5 groups: 10, 20, 40, or 80 mg/day of Policosanol or placebo. No statistically significant difference between Policosanol and placebo was observed.

In none of the secondary outcome measures, namely total cholesterol, HDL, VLDL, triglycerides, lipoprotein(a) and LDL/HDL were there any significant effects of Policosanol.

Recent Internet reviews by WMD dating to February 2015, however, have reported Policosanol to be effective in reducing cholesterol levels. Notably, many of these reviews were provided by people who had suffered intolerable side effects from statins. One such study concluded:

Policosanol has been proven incredibly effective at lowering cholesterol. Study after study (double blind peer reviewed) conducted by both the US government and research centers going back MORE THAN A DOZEN YEARS have definitely proven its effectiveness as well as its lack of negative side effects.

Pectin

Pectin is an amorphous, viscous, water-soluble type of dietary fibre found in fruits and used in making jams and jellies. The main commercial source of pectin is citrus fruit peel. Much of pectin is metabolized by colonic fermentation and slows the rise of blood glucose after a carbohydrate meal. Pectin inhibits LDL peroxidation (Yang et al., 2004), may inhibit LDL synthesis (Westcott, 2002), and lowers cholesterol levels:

(a) In a University of Florida study 15 gm of grapefruit pectin in capsules daily cut TC by 7.6% and LDL by 10.8% (Gottlieb et al, 1990).

(b) 10 gm of pectin daily lowered average cholesterol levels in college students by 20% in just three weeks (Fisher H, *Prevention,* March 1975).

Better still, pectin can reverse atherosclerosis, for example:

(a) Dr James Cerda of U Florida gave miniature pigs 6 to 12 times normal fat intake for 12 months.

Then, with the high-fat diet maintained, he gave half of them 3% grapefruit pectin for a further 9 months, after which he found that the pigs given pectin had 60% less atherosclerosis in their aortas and coronary arteries, regression he thought might be owing to the galacturonic acid of which pectins are a derivative, and independent of the lowering of blood cholesterol levels (Carper, 2000).

(b) A US doctor's father found that taking pectin 3 times daily reduced carotid artery closure from 40% to 25% after 16 months (Carper, 2000).

Pectin helps with arthritis because it smoothes damaged synovial and connective tissue, including arteries, tendons, and ligaments.

Pectin also has a mild chelating effect which, along with improvement in arterial condition, may also help in reversing the progression of vascular disease. Soluble fibre, however, has less cholesterol-lowering effect than other dietary measures (Brown et al., 1999), so the degree to which it can reverse atherosclerosis is also likely to be less.

Normalizing homocysteine levels

According to Carper (2000), experts report that high homocysteine can boost risk of vascular disease as much a fivefold, and heart disease deaths six fold and a 5 year Norwegian study of 900 people confirmed this six fold increase. Even when artery damage is not severe it seems that high homocysteine helps trigger heart attacks.

This is because homocysteine increases protein degradation rates (Sterna et al., 2004), altering the anticoagulant properties of endothelial cells to a procoagulant phenotype (Jacobsen, 1998), making development of plaques and thrombi far more likely.

Digestion of protein produces the amino acid methionine which in turn is converted in steps to homocysteine, cystathionine, and cysteine.

People with the hereditary metabolic disorder *homocystinuria* have a genetic defect in the enzyme cystathionine synthetase, resulting in abnormally high plasma methionine and homocysteine levels, mental retardation, shuffling gait, skeletal deformations and fatal episodic obstruction of blood vessels with clots.

As noted in Chapter 12, homocysteine levels in those not so afflicted can be normalized in 3 months with folic acid (400 mcg) and vitamin B_6 and B_{12} supplementation.

Co-enzyme Q10

For those with serious heart problems Coenzyme Q10 (CoQ10) may be beneficial. CoQ10 is an antioxidant made by the body which is synergistic with vitamins C and E and it also reduces oxidation of cholesterol in blood vessel walls. CoQ10 supplementation is widely used for patients who have suffered heart failure because it reduces shortness of breath and thence hospitalizations. There is, however, no evidence that CoQ10 prevents heart attack or stroke (Cooke & Zimmer, 2002).

Thiamine

Thiamine or vitamin B1 is important for heart function.

Daily dosage of 200 mg for 6 weeks improved left ventricle function in a group of patients in Israel with congestive heart failure (Cooper, 1996).

Twenty-seven inmates of a Malaysian detention centre suffering from ankle swelling and heart problems all showed "prompt, positive clinical response to thiamine replacement therapy" (Cooper, 1996).

Vitamins D and K

Vitamins D (circa 5,000 IU) and K, and phytate (from cereal bran) also prevent vascular calcification (VC). In a 10-year study of 4,800 elderly people, 45 mg/day of K2 [RDI = 70 mcg] halved VC and mortality (Geleijnse et al., *J Nutrition* 2004), whilst extremely high dosages of vitamin K reversed VC in rats[3] by 37% in just six weeks (Schurgers et al., *Blood* 109, 2007, 2823-2831).

Chromium

Studies have shown that chromium supplements lower total cholesterol and LDL and increase HDL. Chromium picolinate has also been found to reduce body fat percentage and increase muscle mass in male athletes.

Lab rats fed a high-sugar, chromium-deficient diet had far more lipid accumulation in their arteries. When chromium was added to the diet cholesterol levels were lowered and there was less arterial lipid accumulation (Lieberman & Bruning, 1997).

Chromium also improves insulin resistance and thus has positive effects on blood sugar and insulin levels, therefore, along with vanadium, being a helpful supplement for combating obesity and type 2 diabetes. (Whitaker, 2002)

The daily chromium intake for the average American is 50-100 mcg, whereas the RDI for chromium is 120 mcg, but long-term studies suggest much more is required to obtain a balance of chromium in the body.

Otherwise adequate diets may be deficient in chromium in part because refining grains removes three quarters of their chromium.

---

[3] Massive IV doses or warfarin are used on lab rats to induce calcification.

Daily supplementation with 400-600 mcg of chromium picolinate or GTF (glucose tolerance factor) chromium is recommended for cholesterol, heart, and diabetes concerns.

A newly discovered antibody 2H10 which can block a protein called Vascular Endothelial Growth Factor (BVEGF-B) may help treat type-2 diabetes. This growth factor affects the transport and storage of fat in body tissue and blocking it helps prevent fat accumulating in damaging places (Julia Medew, 'Promising new drug for diabetes', *The Age,* 27/9/2012).

Magnesium for Prinzmetal's Variant Angina

Considered a newly recognized phenomenon because attacks may occur during sleep (triggered by REM sleep) and are sometimes fatal, variant angina was named for a US doctor circa 50 years ago.

Variant angina can occur at any time during the day as a result of mental or emotional stress, cold weather exacerbating the situation. Some people, for example, find doing fiddly jobs, or doing even routine jobs in haste, can cause heart pain.

Variant angina is caused by *vascular spasm* rather than lack of blood supply to heart muscle because of coronary occlusion. Generally spasm occurs in a section of coronary artery with fatty streaking and close to a significant plaque, perhaps causing moderate (circa 50%) stenosis.

Spasm occurs as a result of acetylcholine induced contraction with (mental) stress. Normally acetylcholine also stimulates endothelial production of NO to dilate the artery again.

When the endothelium is dysfunctional because of either:

(a) A defect in the nitric oxide synthase enzyme, or

(b) Fatty streaking reducing access of NO to the affected artery's smooth muscle cells,

prolonged spasm occurs. This may last a few or several minutes, the pain varying from slight to a crushing pain across the chest

Commonly, calcium channel blockers are prescribed for variant angina but these often cause unpleasant side effects such as headaches. The author, for example, found that Ikorel, the active ingredient of which is the channel blocker nicorandil, made him feel worse not better, whereas magnesium worked well taken either as tablets or very cheap Epsom Salts, the well-known laxative effects of the latter being a reminder of the effectiveness of magnesium as a vasodilator.

Magnesium (dilation) and calcium (contraction) play a fundamental role in muscle function, including that of the smooth muscle cells in arteries.

Not surprisingly, therefore, many people find magnesium supplements the best solution to variant angina problems, one report stating that: "Two studies reported ten years apart indicated that magnesium may be the best treatment for this condition [VA]."

Well-known for reducing arrhythmia, magnesium also dilates coronary vascular tissue, reduces oxidant stress, improves cardiac energy production, reduces platelet aggregation, and regulates heart contractility.

Magnesium also improves conditions of high cholesterol and triglycerides while increasing HDL. In addition, magnesium also modulates synthesis of prostacyclin (Satake et al., 2004).

The RDI for magnesium is 420 mg for males 31-50 but an average diet contains just 300 mg of magnesium, only two-thirds of which is absorbed. Thus for VA, circa 500 mg magnesium is often recommended. Chelated magnesium is much better absorbed, however, and as little as half the dosage of magnesium in this form may be required.

In life-threatening situations, such as after a major heart attack, IV magnesium can be lifesaver and can reduce death rates by 75% (Whitaker, 2002).

The main side effect of magnesium is diarrhea, not surprising as Epsom Salts (magnesium sulphate) have long been taken for constipation, so dosage of magnesium must be limited, but taking smaller amounts two or more times in the day should reduce this side effect.

Other supplements for variant angina

(1) **Taurine.** Levels of the non-essential amino acid taurine tend to become low as we age and 500 - 1000 mg of taurine has been claimed to reduce variant angina, in part because it helps keep potassium and magnesium inside cells while keeping excess sodium out. Taurine is also a potent antioxidant, reduces platelet aggregation, and lowers blood pressure and cholesterol levels.

Both magnesium and taurine have been found to reduce arrhythmia, better results being obtained with both in one study. Taurine has also been used to treat epilepsy and uncontrollable facial twitching, but such applications may require higher dosage.

(2) **Zinc** may also help heart function (Murray, 1977). After only 5 days of a trial of zinc's effect on the common cold,[4] 23 mg zinc lozenges taken every 2 hours caused a man's angina to disappear for the first time in 15 years.

Lower doses have also been found effective, Dr William Halcomb finding that as little as three 60 mg zinc tablets daily (RDI = 14 mg for males 31-50), along with diet changes and quitting smoking, reduced or eliminated the need for nitroglycerin.

(3) **Antioxidants.** Oxy-LDL is the main cause of reduced NO access in VA. Thus antioxidants including C, E and selenium should be included in VA treatment to reduce LDL oxidation.

(4) **Hormones.** When VA occurs in younger people, it is usually in women and progesterone patches have been found to reduce VA spasm in premenstrual women.

Correspondingly, in one study of 62 men with heart disease and low-normal testosterone levels, testosterone patches increased exercise stress test durations before angina onset by 37%, compared to 15% in the placebo group (Whitaker, 2002).

Studies have also found dehydroepaindrosterone (DHEA), a precursor to testosterone and oestrogen, to protect against heart disease (Whitaker, 2002).

A cautionary note, however: US data published online in the journal *Breast Cancer Research* in 2010 showed that a decline in the incidence of breast cancer amongst women over 50 was concentrated in women who had ceased hormone replacement therapy.

Conclusion

Though they could not be more different chemically, Cooke and Zimmer regard NO as a "sister" molecule to prostacyclin because both substances have similar effects upon the blood and its vessels. This was exemplified by the use of another prostaglandin PGE_1 in 1996 to obtain "equivalent" results to those obtained with L-arginine in treating peripheral vascular disease (Cooke and Zimmer, 2002).

---

[4] Studies have found that zinc reduces the severity and duration of colds if given within 48 hours of the onset of symptoms, and that children taking zinc for at least 5 months were less likely to catch a cold.

Thus niacin, fish oils and L-arginine are supplements that can stop the progression of ASHD and even reverse it. To that end, they are taken in combination in the 2-year program of Chapter 30, also including garlic to complement the cholesterol lowering activities of the niacin and fish oils.

In contrast, statins only stabilize plaques to prevent them rupturing to release clots and do not reduce them (Cooke and Zimmer, 2002), but their use as an emergency measure to prevent risk of a second heart attack quickly following a first, for example, might be well advised. In the long term the natural supplements discussed here should also be considered.

To normalize homocysteine levels folic acid + B_6 and B_{12} should also be taken.

Along with iron, B_{12} also helps prevent anaemias, amongst the most easily treatable adverse factors related to heart failure, particularly as the severity of heart failure increases (*Heart, Lung and Circulation* 2010;19;730-735).

Finally, magnesium is highly effective in reducing variant angina and, indeed, may eliminate it for the most part in many cases. Note, however, that alcohol is the most notorious substance for depletion of magnesium in the body, however, another reason for moderation, if not abstention.

Note also that magnesium may be effective in reducing some of the more severe symptoms of PMS and pregnancy such as headaches (Firshein, 1998).

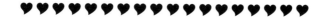

Chapter 14

ANTIOXIDANTS TO PREVENT CARDIOVASCULAR DISEASE

> *Unless those free radicals are neutralized, our risk of suffering more than fifty diseases, including atherosclerosis, heart attacks, various cancers, and cataracts, increases considerably.*
> Dr Kenneth Cooper, *Advanced Nutritional Therapies* (1996).

Introduction

Free radicals play a number of important roles in the body but in excess they can set off a chain reaction of oxidation. Oxidation of LDL cholesterol and other blood lipids contributes to atherosclerosis. Dietary antioxidants supplement the work that enzymes in the body such as superoxide dismutase do to control free radical levels, thereby reducing aging, heart disease and cancer.

Cambridge and Harvard University studies found that 250 - 400 IU of vitamin E daily reduced heart problems by around 40% and Roizen (2000) claims that if the arteries are not fibrotic or permanently hardened vitamin E can reduce heart attack risk by up to 75%.

Artery clogging in monkeys fed a very high fat diet was cut by 60 - 80% when they were also given vitamin E (Carper, 2000). Then with a normal diet and about 100 IU of vitamin E daily artery closure was reduced from 35% to 15% in two years.

Because vitamin C (and E) protect NO (Cooke, 2002), artery dilation of most heart patients given 2000 mg of vitamin C improved by 50% after two hours (Carper, 2000).

Four months after angioplasty to unblock coronary arteries only 24% of patients given 500 mg of vitamin C daily suffered reclosure compared to 43% of the patients not given vitamin C.[1] Thus only 12% of the patients given vitamin C needed further surgery compared to 29% of the patients not given vitamin C.

Vitamin C may also relieve mild hypertension in people of all ages by lowering blood levels of sodium and thus increasing the ratio of potassium to sodium (Gottlieb et al., 1990).

Pomegranate juice, thanks to its antioxidant punicalagins, has been found to have antiatherogenic effects and to reverse arterial disease.

Vitamin E

Antioxidants impede oxidation of LDL particles. Oxidized LDL particles deposited in artery walls become a target for white blood cells which, attempting to protect the body, absorb them and become engorged (Superko, 2004), inflaming the arteries and resulting in the vicious cycle that is atherosclerosis.

The Cambridge Heart Antioxidant Study found that after a first heart attack 400 IU of vitamin E daily almost halved risk of a second (McGowan, 1998). A Harvard University study found that 100 - 250 IU of vitamin E daily for at least two years reduced heart attack incidence by 37 to 41% (Carper, 2000). Another study of over 30,000 physicians found that those who consumed 200 IU of vitamin E daily had 40% fewer heart attacks (Cooke and Zimmer, 2002).

In contrast, the 7-year HOPE-TOO study of 4,000 patients found that vitamin E didn't protect against heart events, instead making hospitalization for heart failure 21% more likely (Lonn et al., 2005).

Vitamin E comes in two forms, tocopherols (the foregoing studies were with these, mostly alpha-tocopherol) and tocotrienols. The latter reduce cholesterol levels and inhibit platelet aggregation, and alpha-tocotrienol has been found to be a 40 - 60 times more powerful antioxidant in inhibiting lipid peroxidation than alpha-tocopherol.

Taking 240 mg of tocotrienols from palm oil for 18 - 36 months has been found to decrease carotid artery plaque (info@tocotrienol.org).

---

[1] Because of the diuretic properties of vitamin C "Its use in heart failure was suggested in 1938 by Evans" (Stone, 1972).

Other antioxidants

The Physician's Health Study of 22,000 doctors aged 40 to 64 found that, in a subgroup of 333 men with histories of heart disease, risk of heart attack, stroke or death was halved in those with an intake of at least 50 mg (approx. 85,000 IU vitamin A) of beta carotene daily. This risk reduction appeared greater than with aspirin but occurred only after 12 months of supplementation (Lieberman & Bruning, 1997; Rath, 2001b).

The Harvard Nurse's Study that tracked 87,000 women nurses for 8 years found that those who ate carrots 5 or more times weekly reduced risk of stroke by 68% compared to those who ate carrots only once a month or less (Carper, 2000).

Belgian researchers found that stroke victims were more likely to survive, have less neurological damage, and to recover completely, if they had above-average levels of vitamin A (Carper, 2000).

In contrast, a controlled trial found that taking 25,000 IU vitamin A for almost 4 years increased triglyceride levels by 11%, cholesterol levels by 3%, and decreased HDL by 1% (Cartmel et al., 1999).

Vitamin C may regenerate other antioxidants like vitamin E (Linus Pauling Institute, 2009) and lack of vitamin C has been shown by research to raise systolic BP by about 16% and diastolic BP by 9% (Carper, 2000).

A UCLA study of the vitamin intake of 11,000 people over 10 years found that if their daily diet had at least 300 mg of vitamin C men had 50% less heart disease and women 40% less (Enstrom, 1992). The study also showed that increased vitamin C uptake increased life expectancy by 6 years, a result contradicted in a later study (Kim, 1994).

A recent US study of 3000 women found that those who took vitamin C reduced stroke risk by 42%. For those who smoked, vitamin C reduced stroke risk by 48% (*The Australian,* 15 Nov. 2006).

Finally, a pooled analysis of the results of many major studies indicated that at least 400 mg vitamin C daily may be required for maximum reduction of heart disease risk (Linus Pauling Institute, 2009).

A study of 454 men aged 40 to 75 who had had a non-fatal heart attack or fatal heart disease compared the results with those from 900 men with no heart disease and found that even after adjusting for diet and lifestyle factors men with vitamin D deficiency had twice the risk of heart attack (Giovanucci et al., *Arch Intern Med* 168 (2008) 1165-1173).

14. Antioxidants to Prevent Cardiovascular Disease

A study of 3258 people who had had angiograms and of whom 22.6% died in the following eight years, found that those with lower levels of vitamin D in their blood were twice as likely to die (Dobnig et al., *Arch Intern Med* 168 (2008) 1340-1349).

Fruit and vegetables are good sources of antioxidants and no doubt this is why a review of studies of 250,000 people who were followed up over an average of 13 years found that eating 3 or more 80g servings of fruit and vegetables a day reduced incidence of strokes by up to 26% (*The Weekend Australian,* 28-29 Jan. 2006).

Red wine contains antioxidants called flavonoids which apparently come from the grape skins and nature has them there to protect the grapes from the sun.

Green tea, however, is one of the most powerful antioxidants but most of this property is lost in dehydration and freezing before export. The solution is green tea extract or pills, if available, or black tea which is also a good antioxidant, though less effective.

Table 14.1 briefly lists some of the best known antioxidants and some of the foods richest in them.

Magnesium bicarbonate is included. This is found in the soils of the Monaro district of that state of New South Wales in Australia. Here livestock were found to live twice as long as normal.

This attracted the interest of a scientist who began selling water laced with magnesium bicarbonate called *Unique Water*. Publicized on TV this product caused quite a stir and there were many reports of almost miraculous results in people with incurable ailments.

Hearing this, the author looked through his research on corrosion of steel reinforcement in concrete (often referred to as 'concrete cancer') done many years earlier. In this work he had concluded that chromate and phosphate compounds were useful as concrete admixtures to prevent reinforcement corrosion or oxidation.

Chromates are toxic, however, so magnesium phosphate, a useful antioxidant, was included in the supplementation program of Chapter 27, in part because magnesium is important in relation to arrhythmia.

Zinc is essential for the synthesis of RNA (ribonucleic acid) and DNA and is also an antioxidant.

Finally, selenium is one of the most important antioxidants but is deficient in the soils and thence foods in some regions. Most doctors, therefore, recommend selenium supplements as well as multivitamin and mineral tablets as a minimum dietary supplementation program.

Table 14.1. Common food sources of the main dietary antioxidants.

Vitamin or mineral	Good food sources	RDI*	Origin*	ODI*
A and beta-carotene	Yellow-orange fruits & vegetables Green, leafy vegetables Carrots	5000 IU	15,000	5,000-50,000
C	Citrus fruits	60 mg	600	500 - 5000
D	Some fish & fish liver oils Fortified no-fat milk 10-20 minutes sun per day	400 IU		400 - 800
E	Vegetable oils, corn, soybean	15 IU	33	400 - 1200
Magnesium phosphate & bicarbonate	Magnesium phosphate in cereals, cocoa & magnesium bicarbonate from soils of certain areas	400 mg (Mg)		500 - 750
Zinc	Sea foods (esp. oysters) Red meats, whole grain foods	15 mg	43	22.5 - 50
Selenium	Sea foods, meat Vegetables from certain regions	75 mcg		50 - 400

* NHMRC 2009, Lieberman & Bruning (1997), Somer (2001).

Table 14.1 shows the RDI's, 'Origin' = estimates of Stone Age man's consumption (Somer, 2001), and optimal daily intakes (ODIs) suggested by Lieberman and Bruning (1997). That RDI for vitamin C is only 10% of the 'origin' intake[2] lends weight to the vitamin C deficiency theory of heart disease, which relies in part on the fact that we have lost the ability to synthesize vitamin C, whereas most animals produce the human equivalent of 1000 mg - 20,000 mg of vitamin C (Rath, 2001b).

This theory is that the lesions that cause atherosclerosis are an early stage of scurvy. Indeed, Passwater (1975) observes that after heart attacks blood vitamin C levels drop to those typical of scurvy.

---

[2] Early humans ate fruits with up to 500 mg of vitamin C daily (Heber, 1998). The RDI for adult males in the USA is now 90 mg (Linus Pauling Inst., 2009).

Other vitamins and minerals

Magnesium is essential for nerve and muscle action and energy metabolism. A ten-year US study of four hundred people who were at high risk of coronary disease found that those who ate a magnesium-rich diet had fewer than half as many complications from cardiovascular-related problems as did those who only ate about one-third of the RDI of magnesium. Overall mortality rates for people who ate a magnesium-rich diet were lower as well.

It has also been known for many years that heart attacks are less common in areas where the water supplies are rich in magnesium.

Magnesium is also known to lower blood pressure, dilate the arteries and help restore normal heart rhythms after a heart attack.

Magnesium also assists in the proper regulation of calcium.

Good food sources are whole grain breads and cereals. Nuts and fruits and vegetables such as bananas, beets, raisins and dates are also good sources.

RDI is 400 mg for women and 333 mg for men.

Potassium is important in the functioning of muscles which contract and relax according to inputs and outputs of calcium and magnesium, potassium playing a part in regulating these ionic flows.

Thus potassium, together with other minerals, regulates blood pressure and helps the heart and kidneys to function property. Several major studies have shown that potassium decreases the incidence of strokes, the major cause of aging of the brain.

One study found that people who had comparatively little potassium had 2.6 to 4.8 times the risk of stroke compared to those who had considerably more potassium. Of 287 people with high potassium intake nobody had a stroke during the study whereas 24 of the 527 people with lower potassium intake had strokes.

Potassium may also prevent other forms of arterial aging. One way in which it does this is thought to be by acting as a counterbalance to sodium intake. Others include stabilization of arterial plaques, decreased oxidation of lipids and stabilization of nerves deprived of oxygen.

Overdosing with potassium can cause problems and supplementation should be avoided. Instead bananas, citrus fruits, dried apricots and peaches, avocados, tomatoes, spinach, celery, sardines, skim milk and low fat yogurt are good sources of potassium. Thus, as always, a well-balanced diet with plenty of fruit and vegetables is recommended.

Conversely, sodium generally needs to be avoided in the diet as it is a major cause of high blood pressure whereas many modern packaged foods and snacks have very high sodium content. Recent findings suggest that excessive sodium intake increases aging. Suggested RDI's are circa 2000 mg but more like 1500 mg is perhaps wiser.

Iron is often recommended, especially for young women with heavy menstruation. Unless you are diagnosed as suffering from iron deficiency anemia, however, you should not need iron supplementation. Indeed, you should avoid it as studies have linked elevated levels to increased incidence of cardiovascular disease and cancer. This is in part because iron forms haemoglobin in the blood and this is an oxidant which increases oxidation of LDL cholesterol, thus causing atherosclerosis.

The role calcium plays in helping prevent osteoporosis, especially in older women, is well known, so much so that the recommended daily intakes of calcium for adult women are 25% higher than for men.

The US National Cancer Institute's bowel cancer prevention web site says that people with diets high in fat, protein, calories, alcohol and both red and white meat, and low in calcium, folate and vitamin D, are more likely to develop colorectal cancer

Vitamin K_2 is formed by bacteria in the large intestine and is associated with reduced likelihood of death, heart disease and severe aortic calcification. Adult vitamin K deficiency is rare but may result from digestive disturbance, perhaps by certain drugs.

Homocysteine interferes with synthesis of collagen and elastin required for healthy arteries. It also irritates arterial linings, causing small lesions which initiate plaques. It may also oxidize LDL, further growing plaques. Excess homocysteine is responsible for 42% of cerebrovascular disease, 30% of cardiovascular disease and 28% of peripheral vascular disease

Taking 400 mcg of folate (folic acid) a day can dramatically reduce homocysteine levels in the blood to acceptable levels within three months.

Folate is one of the B-complex vitamins and is contained in many foods. For example, a glass of orange juice contains 43 mcg but the body absorbs only 50% of folate in food so at least occasional folate supplementation is advisable.

Note too that pregnant women or those somewhat likely to become so should take folic acid supplements (0.4 mg/day) to reduce risk of spina bifida or other neural tube defects in newborns.

Most essential oils have very high ORAC ratings. Sandalwood, tsuga, thyme, grapefruit, frankincense and lemon grass essential oils have been shown to kill up to 90% of cancer cells in vitro. Research published in 2009 showed that low concentrations of linalool, a common essential oil constituent, completely eradicated the HepG2 liver cancer cell line.

Studies have found that 1-15 grams/day of limonene, which is found in a number of essential oils, brought about remission in almost 20% of very advanced cancer patients (Crowell, 1999).

Conclusion

Antioxidants help reduce atherosclerosis and arteriosclerosis. As discussed further in following chapters they also reduce cancer risk.

There have been many conflicting results from trials of the effect of antioxidants on cancer statistics. This is in part because their main effect may be in the early stages whereas it takes up to 14 years for a single breast cancer cell to multiply and produce a tumour large enough to be detectable.

Antioxidants such as vitamin E also reduce aging. This was demonstrated by a study that found that aged mice on a deprived diet were more prone to develop Alzheimer's disease but this trend was reversed when the human equivalent of 2-4 apples a day was added to their diet (*J Alzheimer's Disease* 8 (2006) 283-287).

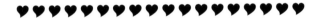

Chapter 15

REDUCING PHYSICAL
& MENTAL AGING

> *The health of your arterial system*
> *is the most important gauge of your Real Age.*
> Michael Roizen, *Real Age* (2000).

Introduction

As noted at the start of Chapter 1, unhealthy arteries not only means development of atherosclerosis, and with it aging of the brain as well, but it also increases cancer risk considerably.

Therefore to reduce both physical and mental aging one should be at pains to establish a sound diet, diet supplement, exercise and relaxation routine along the lines discussed in earlier chapters to normalize cholesterol and homocysteine levels, including plenty of antioxidants to reduce DNA mutations and thence cancer risk.

A truly healthy lifestyle will also reduce the effects of any harmful food substances and any genetic disadvantages you may have concerning, for example, predisposition to heart disease or breast cancer.

Antioxidants to improve IQ in the young

Dr A.C. Kubala et. al. divided 351 students into two groups, those with higher, and those with lower vitamin C levels. Those with higher C levels were 4.5 points higher in IQ (Holford, 2009).

In another study, Patrick Holford, Stephen Schoenhaler, John Yudkin, Hans Eysenck and Linus Pauling gave 30 children a special multivitamin and mineral supplement and 30 others a placebo.

After 8 months of the supplement children's average non-verbal IQ[1] was 10 points higher, with some children being up to 20 points higher. Several other studies have had similar findings.

Another study of 200 teenagers in Dakota found that 20 mg (but not 10mg, the RDI being 7 mg) of zinc increased memory accuracy and attention spans (Holford, 2009).

Contrastingly, MIT researchers found that children with diets high in refined carbohydrates such as sugar, white bread and sweets, had IQ up to 25 points lower (Schauss, 1983).

Some of the studies that have made such findings have sometimes included infants, improved IQ from diet improvements showing up a few years down the track. Thus, pregnant women would be wise to ensure that their diets are as healthy as possible and include some of the key nutrients discussed in this chapter.

Thus, as might be expected, a healthy diet with appropriate vitamin and mineral supplements will help reduce age-related memory loss.

Aging of the skin

When we age our most, if not all, of our body's many processes become less efficient. A case in point is that of usage of vitamin C for which the RDA is far too low at only about 10% of what our hunter-gatherer forefathers consumed. Vitamin C is vital for collagen production and, short of it, various structures of our body deteriorate and become softer and the skin decreases in quality, dries out, and wrinkles more and more, covering as it does now more spongy, less muscular tissues beneath, now that our testosterone levels have been falling gradually since about age 20 in males, and ditto perhaps in females.

In older women, however, plentiful fatty adipose tissue disguises the loss of muscle somewhat, if not a lot, though its generally only those not very fat women that reach really old age, that is into their 90s these days.

What to do? Vitamin E creams were all the go 2 or 3 decades ago but now a huge range of skin care products is available, from moisturizers to makeup for whatever skin colour you aspire to. Some of these, particularly those claiming anti-aging properties will contain a host of antioxidants from a variety of sometimes relatively rare and exotic plant sources.

---

[1] Non-verbal IQ is more fluid and susceptible to brain chemistry, while the verbal IQ is more influenced by teaching.

If you can afford these products OK, if not get your weight under control and develop a healthy lifestyle and include plenty of antioxidant rich foods in your diet, adding supplemental antioxidants like beta-carotene, C and E as well.

Then a little red wine rich in procyanidins, or dark grape juice for its resveratrol, or pomegranate juice for its punicalagins, will be helpful in reducing aging of the body both within and on the surface.

For men beards and constant shaving thereof does nothing for the skin but now there are moisturizing products for men that might help a bit, or even fairly cheap Sorbolene will help the skin a little, for example spread on those eyelids which begin to droop with age.

If desperate one can resort to various kinds of surgery to reduce aging, including injection of filler substances to fill out the tissues below wrinkled facial skin. The focus of this book, however, is largely neutraceutical, not surgical.

Finally, don't forget the SPF sunscreen when out and about on higher UV level days.

Macular degeneration

Macular degeneration is one of many diseases of old age, one that is the most common cause of blindness in people over 50. Its cause is not clear as yet, but one theory is that the membrane that separates the eye's photoreceptors from their blood supply develops fatty deposits that interfere with the supply of nutrients.

A Harvard study found that higher blood levels of homocysteine made age-related macular degeneration (AMD) more likely, concluding that AMD and heart disease had some causes in common (Seddon, 2006). Not surprisingly, therefore, a study by the US National Eye Institute found that people taking high levels of antioxidants reduced their risk of developing advanced macular degeneration by 25 per cent.

New laser therapies also promise to slow or reverse age-related macular degeneration (*The Herald Sun,* Melbourne, Nov. 9, 2012).

Memory loss with age

Jane Durga at Wageningen University in the Netherlands gave 818 people aged 50-75 800 mg of folic acid (about 3 times the RDA) a day, or a dummy pill. Three years later the supplement users did as well as people 5.5 years younger on memory tests, and as well as people 1.9 years younger on cognitive speed tests (Holford, 2009).

As this improvement no doubt related to reduction of homocysteine levels, homocysteine being one of the main villains in both atherosclerosis and neural pathway deterioration, other homocysteine-lowering nutrients such as B6 and B12 should be likely to reduce brain aging as well and, indeed, studies are in progress on this issue (Holford, 2009).

As noted in the previous section, antioxidants improve IQ in children. They also reduce memory loss with aging, much of which is owing to reduced liver function, and antioxidants reduce the 'detox burden' on the liver (which may include excess alcohol).

Well-known now, DHA and EPA oils improve brain function.

The herb ginkgo biloba is also helpful and a double-blind placebo-controlled French trial found that giving 320 mg a day to 60 to 80 year-olds improved cognitive processing speed to that of healthy young adults (Holford, 2009).

Acetyl-L-carnitine (ACL) boosts energy production in the brain, improves the brain's glutamate receptors which are responsible for learning, and may stop formation of lipofucian, an "age spot" in neurons that interferes with memory (Gottlieb, 2000).

ACL is expensive, however, and glutamine, the most abundant amino acid in the cerebrospinal fluid surrounding the brain, is an alternative. One US study of healthy volunteers found glutamine enhanced problem-solving ability in continuous performance tests.

Last, but not least, as noted in Chapter 13, phospholipids are also helpful in reducing age-related problems.

Acetylycholine is derived from phosphatidylcholine or pure lecithin[2] and deficiency of this is probably, after high homocysteine levels, the main cause of declining memory with age, and Holford (2009), who calls acetylcholine "the memory molecule," recommends 5 to 10 gm of (commercial) lecithin to maximize mental function.

---

[2] See section 1 of Chapter 2 for the composition of commercial lecithin.

Gottlieb notes that 300 mg/day of another phospholipid, phosphatidyl serine (PS), has been found to reverse the chronological age of the outside layers of neurons by up to 12 years (Gottlieb, 2000).

Thus, to combat memory loss with age take[3]:

➢ Folic acid and B12, and also B6 and B1, B2, B3.
➢ Lecithin [5 - 10 gm], phosphatidyl choline (pure lecithin) or phosphatidyl serine. As noted in Chapter 2, linseeds will help absorption of lecithin.
➢ 1000 mg DHA and EPA, i.e. two fish oil capsules.
➢ Antioxidants A, C [3 gm], E [100 IU/decade of age], selenium and zinc.
➢ Glutamine [5 - 10 gm].
➢ Ginkgo biloba, 160 – 320 mg.
➢ Acetyl-L-carnitine (ACL), 250 – 2,000 mg.

Finally, sustained stress is harmful to the brain[4] so relaxation and exercise (including mental exercise) will help reduce memory loss with age.

Alzheimer's Disease

Supplements required for this are, of course, similar to those of the preceding section:

➢ Folic acid [10 mcg], B12 [250 mcg] and B6 [20 mg] to reduce homocysteine levels.
➢ Lecithin (+ linseeds for absorption) to provide phospholipids. Firshein (1998) recommends phosphatidyl serine dosage of 150-300 mg/day.
➢ Omega-3 from fish oils.
➢ Turmeric contains anti-inflammatory curcumin which breaks up plaques in Alzheimer's patients' brains (Holford, 2009).
➢ Antioxidants as in the preceding section.
➢ DHEA [15 mg], a precursor to testosterone and oestrogen.
➢ N-acetyl cysteine which is converted into the brain's primary antioxidant glutathione.
➢ Hyperzia serrata [200 mg], a moss which helps keep the neurotransmitter acetylcholine in circulation.
➢ Acetyl-L-carnitine (ACL), 500 – 2,000 mg/day.

---

[3] Daily dosages recommended by Holford (2009) shown in [ ] brackets.
[4] Because the stress hormone cortisol shrinks dendrites (Holford, 2009).

Parkinson's Disease

The conventional treatment for Parkinson's disease is the drug L-dopa which is a direct precursor of dopamine.

As with Alzheimer's, also a neural issue, homocysteine levels are linked to Parkinson's and B6 plays an additional role independent of its homocysteine-lowering one in preventing Parkinson's.

Indeed, Geoffrey and Lucille Leader tested patients with Parkinson's and found that "literally 100 percent of them had nutritional deficiencies based on tests that measure what is going on in the cells" (Holford, 2009).

Antioxidants help prevent free-radical damage to brain cells, slowing progression of Parkinson's disease, a 7-year pilot study finding that 3 gm C and 3,200 IU of E delayed the need for drug therapy by up to 2 or 3 years (Holford, 2009). This study used alpha-tocopherol; much better results would be expected with the more potent tocotrienol forms of E.

Coenzyme Q10 is also helpful, being one of the most important antioxidants for protecting mitochondria, and a US study of 80 patients found that 1200 mg of CoQ10 slowed loss of motor function by 44%, 300-600 mg slowing it by 20% (Holford, 2009). ⟵ubiquinol (not ubiquinone)

Thus useful supplements for Parkinson's disease include:

➤ B6, folic acid and B12. ⟵ methylated
➤ CoQ10 [1200 mg].
➤ Magnesium.
➤ C [3 gm], E [3,200 IU], selenium and zinc.

Plenty of protein should also be had, perhaps some of it as supplements, because protein is converted with the aid of B6 to L-phenylalanine. This, with the aid of folate, magnesium, manganese, iron, copper, zinc and C, is converted to L-tyrosine which the same substances convert to L-dopa which is for conventional drug treatment (Holford, 2009).

B6 and zinc then convert L-dopa to dopamine, C converts this to noradrenalin, which B12, folate and niacin then convert to adrenalin.

It also helps to reduce stress levels, avoid environmental and other toxins, and reduce auto-intoxication from constipation by taking magnesium, perhaps as cheap Epsom Salts, magnesium also being helpful for muscle, arterial and brain function.

Finally, according to Gottlieb (2000) Parkinson's patients have low levels of the hormone DHEA (dehydroepaindrosterone) and medically supervised supplementation (10 mg/day for women and 25 mg/day for men) may reduce symptoms.

Multiple sclerosis

Homocysteine attacks arteries and causes of atherosclerosis, but also attacks nerves and neural pathways in the brain. Many of the supplements cited in this chapter should be helpful in treating MS, in particular B12, injections of which totally eliminated symptoms in one patient (Firshein, 1998) and perhaps vitamin D now being trialed for MS treatment. Low fat diets have also "consistently shown significant reduction in relapse rates and slowing of disease progression" for MS (Jelinek, 2010), whilst stress reduction may also be helpful (Kalb, Holland & Giesser 2007).

Mental illnesses

Many of the supplements noted in earlier sections are helpful with mental illnesses, including B-vitamins, vitamin C, phospholipids, fish oils, magnesium, and zinc. Several other supplements are also helpful, including niacin, manganese, and chromium (Holford, 2009).

Hormone treatments

Every woman has heard of HRT after menopause and, equally, men can benefit from extra hormones. With less efficiency of body processes it is difficult to put on muscle at 60+ but hormone supplements and exercise routines for muscle building will help.

Osteoporosis

Another affliction of decaying older people, this can be ameliorated by taking 600 – 1500 mg calcium, 600 mg magnesium to maintain a balance between Ca and Mg, and 400 IU D/day (Gottllieb, 2000).

Note too that exercise will help maintain stronger bones whilst a sound atherosclerosis-combating lifestyle will reduce arterial calcification and thence reduce the amount of calcium stolen from bones for this purpose, a double benefit.

Conclusion

Sound programs for diet and diet supplements including plenty of antioxidants, exercise, and relaxation will all help combat some of the key causes of aging, that is, reduced immune function, atherosclerosis, deterioration of collagen and thence skin, and DNA mutations.

B vitamins, phospholipids, fish oils, antioxidants, amino acids, glutamine, magnesium, hormones, turmeric, ginkgo and hyperzia serrata help deal with neurological problems, along with sound diet, exercise and stress reduction regimes.

Finally, thinking young won't hurt, along with plenty of continuing learning to keep the brain in some sort of shape. Indeed, in this context I calculate 'real IQ' (RIQ) as

Latent IQ $- a$(defects) $+ b$(yrs learning) $+ c$(creativity) $- d$ |age -18|

the last term a Heavyside step function and b not constant (Mohr, 2014; Mohr et al., 2017) but circa 1 in teenage years and more like 0.5 perhaps in later life, whereas for decline d could be assumed to be about 0.25.

Taking a hypothetical example, a top of the class student at 18 might have IQ = 140 at that age but one can increase this with further learning by studying, say, for 5 years, at which point the persons real IQ can be estimated as RIQ = 140 + 0.5(5) − 0.25(5) = 141.25.

This is not a big increase, but at least it's not the usual decline. Then if this person goes into serious research, is careful with diet etc., as discussed earlier, then at age 48 the calculation may become something like:

RIQ = 180 + 30(0.5) − 30(0.25) = 147.5

which is a worthwhile improvement indeed!

I shan't worry about coefficient a at this point as it might vary for different types of genetic defects that result from problems such as Fragile X and Down's syndromes, and, of course, degrees of mental retardation can fall into four classes:

➤ Mild.
➤ Moderate.
➤ Severe.
➤ Profound.

Then there are external influences such as malnutrition, lead poisoning and fetal alcohol syndrome, to name just a few. Depressive illnesses, even being slave to a lousy, bullying boss could be a factor.

Finally, as noted earlier in this chapter, such substances as lecithin, magnesium fish oils, zinc, and vitamins A, B-group, C, D and E are helpful in improving brain function, especially in the very young and the very old (Holford & Colson, 2008).

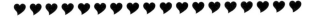

Chapter 16

THE 10% FAT CALORIES SOLUTION

> *I have had numerous discussions with physicians who*
> *acknowledge that 10 percent calories from fat*
> *is the optimal level, but then they go on to say something*
> *along the lines of "My patients would never accept - " .*
> Raymond Kurzweil, *The 10% Solution For A Healthy Life:*
> *How to Eliminate Virtually All Risk of Heart Disease and Cancer* (1993).

Fad diets

The diet 'minefield' is difficult enough to navigate without the plethora of fad diets that we have seen in modern times.

In the 1930s a number of vogue diets were based on acid/alkaline ideas with little medical basis (Varona, 2001). As noted in Chapter 3 and the last chapter, however, it is important for diet to be reasonably neutral on the pH scale as excessive acidity reduces cellular oxygen levels and thus encourages tumour growth.

The Atkins "super energy diet" (1978) advocates plenty of fat to give you energy, arguing that you will be energized and burn it up easily and that in most cases people won't even need to keep track of their calorie intake. Atkins limits carbohydrate, on the other hand, especially sugar which he describes as *"the world's most dangerous food additive."*

To lose weight Atkins suggests limiting carbohydrate intake to 10 grams daily, an impossibly small amount. To maintain weight he suggests 60 grams and to gain weight he suggests 100 grams, still a quite small amount. Today we deal with the carbohydrate question by encouraging low GI foods.

In an earlier book (1973) he says we can eat "any kind of meat in any quantity - except meat with fillers such as sausage, hot dogs, meatballs, most packaged 'cold cuts'." This flies in the face of modern thinking on saturated fat.

In a study of 20 obese men and women half had a low-fat diet, and half a low-carb diet for six weeks, after which ultrasound measurements showed that the low-fat diet gave improved artery expansion, whereas the low-carb one gave reduced artery expansion, an early sign of heart disease typical of excessive fat intake (Phillips SA et al., *Hypertension* 51 (2008) 376-382).

The "Zone" diet advocates a dietary calorie breakdown of 40% carbohydrate, 30% protein and 30% fat (Sears, 1995). It is claimed that this gives a balance of "good" and "bad" eicosanoids, "superhormones" that control other hormones such as insulin and glucagon.

It is also claimed that: *Virtually every disease state - - whether it be heart disease, cancer, or autoimmune diseases like arthritis and multiple sclerosis - - can be viewed at the molecular level as the body simply making more bad eicosanoids and fewer good ones.*

The Zone Diet has been found to work well for elite athletes, no doubt in part because it is high in protein and in part because eicosanoid balance optimizes the ability to burn up stored carbohydrate and protein rapidly.

For most of us, however, the unused protein will simply be stored as fat in the long run and Cooper (1996) suggests 10-20% of calories as protein whilst Corder suggests 20% as optimal (2007).

During WWII "strenuous efforts were made in Britain and Europe - - - to keep the fat content of diet as high as possible" because it was felt the if dietary fat fell below 25% of calories people accustomed to much more than this would suffer gastric distress (Clements & Rogers, 1967).

In those days, indeed, the only recommendations about macronutrient intake limits (carbohydrate, fat and protein) concerned minimum protein requirements which were 70 gm for a 70 kg person (Clements & Rogers, 1967), a figure arrived at in 1922 and subsequently adopted by the WHO (Steele, 1985).

More recently most authorities suggest no more than 30% fat calories (Stanton, 1984). From what we know now, however, 30% fat calories is just too much for those of us concerned about heart disease or cancer.

The Pritikin weight loss diet (1981) advocates plenty of complex carbohydrates from whole grains, vegetables and fruits but cautions against refined sugar and restricts calories heavily to from 700 to 1200 daily.

The F-Plan diet (Eyton, 1982) recommends 35-50 gm of fibre daily and the diet programs of Chapter 17 provide satisfactory fibre intake.

The 10% solution

Kurzweil (1993) advocates a 10% fat calories limit to *"virtually eliminate all risk of cancer and heart disease"* and backs this claim up with masses of WHO epidemiological evidence from around the world.

In contrast, recent studies using diets with 20% fat calories found little reduction in cancer and heart disease (*AMA J* 295 (2006) 629-4, 643-66).

The Ornish diet (1996) also advocates a 10% fat calories limit, and Christensen (2001) suggests that this "aggressive" limit is appropriate for a sedentary 60 year old man with CHD and a history of chest pain diagnosed as stable angina.

In a five-year study an experimental group following the Ornish program of low-fat, whole-foods, vegetarian diet, aerobic exercise, and stress management training showed continued regression of arterial blockages and reduced LDL by 40% in one year, maintaining half this reduction at the end of five years.

The control group, despite some of them receiving cholesterol-lowering drugs and some bypass surgery, deteriorated during the same period.

A further 3-year study of a control group of 139 and a group of 194 candidates for heart surgery following Ornish's program gave remarkable results.

The 194 heart surgery candidates all improved their blood lipid levels modestly (TC 202→183, LDL 123→102, HDL 37→42, TG 230→201), lost weight and 150 were able to avoid surgery during the 3 year program.

If one is able to achieve the cholesterol reductions of Tables 12.1 and 12.3, therefore, one might indeed feel even more confident of reversing heart disease and minimizing the risk of cancer. This is the objective of this book.

A case study

McGowan's book (1998) gives an excellent case study of a man whose father and mother had died of heart attacks at the ages of 52 and about 60 respectively. At age 30 the man's total cholesterol level was found by a routine test to be 253, considered average at the time.

Soon afterwards his BP was found to be high and medication prescribed. He embarked on a solid exercise program to reduce his weight and BP and get off the medication.

A little over a decade later he began feeling chest pressure. It got worse and after a few weeks he was put into hospital for a week after a heart attack. His weight and BP were ideal and his total cholesterol (TC) level was a good 168. Just as with periods of great stress, this level rises before a heart attack and drops for a month or two later. Worse still, his HDL was not measured and he was told his symptoms were all caused by stress.

A few months later he changed physician and was put on medication which made little difference and he was unable to walk half a block without pain. At age 58 he surrendered to surgery and a bypass operation. A year later he met Mary McGowan and his cholesterol readings were as shown in the first column of results in Table 16.1.

Table 16.1. Cholesterol results, mg/dL (McGowan, 1998).

	Initial	8 weeks	20 weeks	32 weeks	Desirable
TC	181	188	207	169	< 200
LDL	105	115	109	109	< 100
HDL	25	34	31	39	> 45
TC/HDL	7.3	5.5	6.7	4.3	< 4
Triglycerides	247	193	251	104	< 150

His chest pains had discouraged, if not prevented, exercise and he was now 11 kilos overweight, in turn resulting in a high triglyceride level and low HDL. With the aim of weaning him off his BP medication he was given a diet and exercise program.

Eight weeks later he had lost nearly 7 kilos and was still taking his BP medication but less of it. Now his TC/HDL ratio had improved and he wanted more time on his diet and exercise program rather than take medication for his cholesterol levels.

After 20 weeks, however, his ratio had deteriorated because of a few Christmas parties but he insisted on continuing his diet and exercise program for a further twelve weeks rather than take medication.

After 32 weeks his cholesterol profile was almost satisfactory and his BP medication dosage had been further reduced.

The persistent patient's key to success had been many ideas for diet and exercise improvement and, with patience, he obtained a satisfactory cholesterol profile without medication, unusual for somebody with a long history of elevated cholesterol levels, chest pains, and BP medication that reduces HDL, not to speak of fairly recent bypass surgery.

A major key to the improved results in Table 16.1 was McGowan's recommended 20% fat calories limit. The results are, nevertheless, only modest improvements, LDL still being a little high and HDL a little too low. Much better results are obtained with a 10% fat calories limit.

The 10% fat calories limit

Table 16.2. Kurzweil's cholesterol lowering results, mg/dL.

	June 1987	October 1988	January 1989
% fat calories	40%	30%	10%
exercise calories per week	800	1,200	2,000
Total cholesterol	234	193	110
LDL		94	57
HDL	27	28	44
Triglycerides	616	354	43
TC/HDL	8.7	6.9	2.5
weight (lbs)	185	185	160
% heart risk	175	143	5

Raymond Kurzweil's father had died quite young of a sudden heart attack. Himself, finding the 30% fat calorie limit suggested by a doctor had not obtained the desired results, he decided to follow the Pritikin diet guideline of 10% fat calories. The results he obtained in three months are shown in the Table 16.2.

The results are impressive and it is the 10% fat calories limit, along with exercise and watching total calories in order to lose weight, that Kurzweil (1993) recommends as the key to reversing vascular disease and greatly reducing risk of heart attack, stroke and cancer.

Note, however, that at least 5% of calories should be fat to provide enough fat for the body, for example to maintain cell membranes and endothelium linings, and to provide energy for brain and other functions.

Comparing cholesterol reduction results

Table 16.3. Cholesterol reduction results, mg/dL.

Program	1	2		3		4	
Duration	8 weeks	14 weeks		60 weeks		12 weeks	
Results	Change	Before	After	Before	After	Before	After
TC	-31.7%	251	155 (-38%)	234	193 (-18%)	193	110 (-43%)
LDL	-47.5%	172	84 (-51%)			94	57 (-39%)
HDL	+60.6%	41	48 (+17%)	27	28 (+4%)	28	44 (+57%)
TG	-42.1%	191	116 (-42%)	616	354 (-43%)	354	43 (-88%)

Table 16.3 summarizes the results obtained in four cholesterol reduction programs.

Briefly, these involved:

(1) 3 gm niacin daily, fat calories limit of 30%, moderate exercise, and oat-bran muffins had 2 or 3 times daily (Kowalski, 1988). Results are for 12 trial patients with good program compliance.

(2) 2.5 gm niacin daily, fat calories limit of 20% and moderate exercise (McGowan, 1998). Results are for one patient.

(3) 30% fat calories limit and 1200 exercise calories per week (Kurzweil, 1993).

(4) 10% fat calories limit and 2000 exercise calories per week (Kurzweil, 1993).

Programs (3) and (4) were consecutive and for Kurzweil himself.

The results clearly show:

(a) That high dosage niacin substantially improves cholesterol profiles.

(b) That Kurzweil's "10% solution" does even better, whereas with a 30% fat limit results are poor except for a substantial triglyceride (TG) reduction. Notably, Kurzweil lost no weight in (3) but 25 pounds in (4) with a 10% fat calories limit.

McGowan (1998) cites a further patient for whom high dose niacin improved cholesterol levels substantially. Furthermore, after a little over a year, blockage in the circumflex branch of his left coronary artery was reduced from 85% to 65%, a spectacular result that must have resulted more from 'relaxation' of the artery than from reduction in atheroma.

As for diet, Borushek and Borushek (1981) claim that appropriate diet often reduces [total and LDL] cholesterol levels by 10 - 20% in 2 - 4 weeks, and by up to 25% in 6 - 8 weeks.

McGowan (1998), for example, cites the case of a patient with a TG reading above 2600 and HDL of 17 because of high sugar consumption. With simple diet changes, his levels were 298 and 24 only a month later.

Better still, Cooke and Zimmer (2002) note that a 10% fat calories limit can slow and even reverse coronary artery narrowing.

Most studies, of course, have single-mindedly involved one particular dietary supplement or restriction along with a little exercise.

Cooke and Zimmer (2002), for example, focus on high dosage L-arginine in conjunction with a so-called 'Mediterranean diet' which involves a much too liberal 34% of calories from fat.

The importance of exercise in improving lipid levels is exemplified well by a case study cited by Murray (1977) in which, after 4 sedentary days, 7 hyperlipidemic men were made to run 3 or 4 miles in 40 minutes on 4 successive days. Their triglyceride levels on days 4 - 8 were: 235, 173, 136, 119, 104,

an excellent example of how exercise rapidly reduces triglyceride and thence other blood lipid levels.

iological results

Kurzweil's book *The 10% Solution for a Healthy Life* (1993) used large amounts of World Health Organization data to establish by 'line of best fit to the data analysis' the following formulas for the risk of heart disease with increasing values of C = ratio of total cholesterol to HDL level:

Risk for men = 1.357 ln(C) - 1.1875

Risk for women = 2.069 ln(C) - 2.042

where ln( ) = natural logarithm. For example, a man with an acceptable total cholesterol level TC = 180 and a good HDL level = 60 has C = 3 and therefore risk = 0.30 or 30% of the average risk.

On the other hand a man with TC = 240, once deemed acceptable (just!), and HDL = 20 (levels almost this low are common) has C= 12 and thence risk = 2.18 or more than double the average risk.

Kurzweil's book also gives graphs of World Health Organization data for the incidence of three types of cancer in various countries of the world plotted against their average daily fat consumption F gm/day. Lines of best fit for cancer death rates per 100,000 people (R) were:

Breast cancer: R = 24(F - 30)/130
Colon cancer: R = 24(F - 30)/150
Prostate cancer: R = 16(F - 30)/130

30g or less per day

Here F = 30 gives zero (in reality minimal) risk.
Then for F = 60 colon cancer risk is R = 24(60 - 30)/150 = 4.8
If fat consumption doubles to F = 120, then
R = 24(120 - 30)/150 = 14.4

and colon cancer risk has tripled.

This is because high-fat diets create a hospitable environment for anaerobic bacteria in the large intestine. Such bacteria can convert intestinal bile acids into carcinogenic acids. Apparently, weak acids like vitamin C inhibit this process.

To minimize cancer risk Kurzweil recommends limiting fat intake to 10% of total calories. Noting that 1 gm of fat produces 9 calories of energy 'zero risk' F = 30 gm gives 270 calories. If this is 10% of total calories then total calories will be 2700 calories, a reasonable amount for a moderately active young adult male (Borushek, 2014).

Kurzweil's findings are supported by the Australian National Health and Medical Research Council which says that 66 to 75 per cent of bowel cancer cases could be prevented by eating a healthy low fat, high fibre diet with plenty of vegetables and exercising regularly.

Note that excess sugar and protein in the diet will be stored as body fat if not used. Note also that the important role which glucose plays in cancer is emphasized by the success of new chemotherapy drugs that kill cancer cells by blocking their glucose metabolism.

Kurzweil goes on to point out that, although two out of three Japanese men smoke, the incidence of lung cancer in Japan is the lowest in the industrialized world and the incidence of heart disease is also very low because the Japanese diet is low in fat.

Kurweil's figures suggest part of the reason why the Moerman cancer therapy of low fat diet and high supplementation in vitamins A, C and E was found to cure vascular disease, namely that its very low fat intake reduces cholesterol levels (Jochems, 1990, Mohr, 2012b, 2013).

The effect of fat overdoses

Fats are a key part of the cell membranes but saturated fat makes cell membranes stiffer, stiffer cells in the smooth muscle cells of the arteries making them less responsive to blood flow. Saturated fat also makes the arteries walls sticky, reducing blood flow further.

Cooke and Zimmer (2002) note that a meal high in saturated or trans fats raises blood fat levels significantly just two hours later and can damage the endothelium within hours.

One study found that a meal with one gram of saturated fat per kg of body weight increased artery inflammation and reduced artery flexibility, whereas a meal with the same amount of polyunsaturated fat did not have the same negative results (SJ Nicholls et al., *J Amer Coll Cardiology*, 48 (2006) 715-720).

Another study found that a high fat meal caused brachial artery flexibility to deteriorate to about half normal (Cooke and Zimmer, 2002).

Another reason to avoid processed, fried and fast food is that, besides saturated fat aplenty, they contain particularly atherogenic *oxycholesterol.*

Encouraging reverse cholesterol transport

The ultimate aim of a low fat diet is to prevent or even reverse progression of atherosclerosis. Low total blood lipid levels but high HDL levels will increase reverse cholesterol transport (RCT) from macrophages by forcing consequently lipid-poor HDL to desorb cholesterol from plaques by efflux by passive diffusion according to the concentration gradient, assisted by ABCA1 (a transmembrane protein), caveolins (cholesterol-binding proteins), and sterol-27 hydroxylase.

Then the now mature HDL can absorb additional cholesterol via efflux mediated by ABCG1 and SR-B1 (scavenger receptor B1) and carry it to the liver for breakdown into bile acids for excretion (Lewis and Rader, 2005; Ohashi et al., 2005).

RCT is also aided by enzymes such as lecithin-cholesterol acyltransferase (LCAT) and phospholipid transfer protein (PTP).

Regression with low-fat diet and exercise

How experimental high fat diets quickly caused atherosclerosis in lab animals was discussed in Chapter 1. A spectacular example, Dr Draga Vesselinovitch at the University of Chicago obtained a 50% reduction of artery damage in monkeys after 18 months of low-fat diet, with blockages regressing and artery condition improving (Whitaker, 2002).

Nathan Pritikin was one of the pioneers of the 10% fat limit.

Another was Dean Ornish with his Lifestyle Heart Program at UCLA. He gave 23 patients a 24-day in-hospital lifestyle program. Angiography showed they had at least 50% blockage of at least one coronary artery and they were having an average of 10 angina attacks per week

After 24 days on an ultra-low fat vegetarian diet, also practicing stress reduction techniques, their cholesterol dropped by an average of 20.5% and there was a 91% decrease in the frequency of angina, attacks being reduced to just one a week from 10.

A one-year trial with 28 patients followed. This also included moderate exercise and quitting smoking. At the end, compared to a control group of 20 with standard medical care, cholesterol levels fell by 24.3% and LDL by 37.4%, an excellent result *without drugs.*

There was a 91% reduction in angina frequency, along with 28% reduction in severity and 42% reduction in duration.

Average blockage decreased from 40% to 37.8% with improvement greater in the more severely blocked arteries. In contrast, blockage increased significantly in the control group.

A 5-year lifestyle study followed in which the control group endured twice as many heart attacks and heart operations.

A spectacular case study was that of a 61 year-old man who had had angina for 13 years and two of his coronary arteries had 75% and 95% blockage. Rather than have a bypass op, he increased his daily walking from 2 miles to 6. Then he started slow jogging and his angina disappeared in 2 months, and he maintained his program for 7 years, reducing his two artery blockages to 30% and 50%, an excellent result.

Conclusion

Cholesterol normalization can be achieved by diet (with modest levels of supplementation) and exercise and without medication.

If you do have concerns or symptoms of any kind, however, you should see your physician for advice.

As a beginning, have your cholesterol levels checked. Total level can be checked in a few minutes at pharmacies but you should also have your LDL, HDL, Lp(a) and triglyceride levels checked too.

Note that some people with LDL pattern A, that is mainly large LDL particles, suffer an increase in small dense LDL (SDL) when on low fat diets (i.e., 20% fat calories) so it may be worth checking apolipoprotein B level as this indicates SDL level. In such cases niacin or other cholesterol lowering supplements may be required. People with LDL pattern B, or a predominance of SDL, however, do benefit from low fat diets, and these are the people most prone to heart disease (Superko, 2004).

Ultra-low fat diets (≤ 10% fat calories) should benefit people with LDL patterns A and B as these reduce all types of 'bad' cholesterol.

Finally, for those with a family history of early onset of heart disease and cancer the Mohr Plan will definitely reduce their risk of these illnesses considerably. Genetic disposition to small dense LDL, for example, can be handled just by weight watching and restricting saturated fat and simple sugars. Similarly, we inherit one of types E2, E3, E4 of the apolipoprotein E gene from each parent, E3 being normal and E2 and E4 mutations. People with the E2/2 combination are prone to type 3 hyperlipidaemia and thus tuberoeruptive xanthomas or marbles of fat under the skin and also in the arteries. This condition can be controlled by low-calorie diet that avoids sugar as far as possible (Superko, 2004).

16. The 10% Fat Calories Solution

Chapter 17

DEVELOPING A DIET
TO MINIMIZE RISK

> *A landmark Dutch study found that eating, on average,*
> *a mere ounce of fish a day cut the chances*
> *of fatal heart disease by half.*
> Jean Carper, *The Miracle Heart* (2000).

The diet plan

Developing a diet to minimize aging and the risk of heart disease should involve the following objectives:

[1] Remove saturated fat from the diet

This can be done relatively easily, for example by:

(a) Using only skim milk which, fortunately, contains roughly the same amount of calcium.

(b) Eating meat rarely, if at all. Such products as bacon, sausages, meat pies and dim sims are high in saturated fats and cholesterol.

(c) Substituting fish for meat - it has been claimed that eating fish once a week almost halves risk of sudden death.

(d) Avoiding cheese, except perhaps for very low fat cheese only occasionally.

(e) Take special care to avoid high-fat snack foods such as potato crisps, corn chips or cheesy snacks. If you do have such things, 'once in a blue moon' then have only those that are labeled 97% fat free or cooked in olive oil, and these may also have less salt.

(f) Avoid chocolate, except perhaps for dark chocolate only rarely as this has the saving grace of being relatively high in antioxidants.

(g) Avoid high-fat baked goods such as cakes and doughnuts.

(h) Replace saturated fats with mono- and polyunsaturated fats and oils by using canola and olive oil based margarines and cooking with canola, olive, sunflower, soybean and rice oils.

[2] Increase fibre in the diet

A study of 10,469 physicians between the years 1982 and 2006 found that those who ate whole-grain breakfast cereal daily were 28% less likely to develop fatal heart disease compared to those who never ate whole-grain breakfast cereal (L Djoussé et al., *Circulation,* vol. 115, 2007). In this study breakfast cereals were classified as wholegrain if they contained at least 25% oats or bran.

A healthy diet therefore, begins with a high-fibre bran cereal for breakfast and includes wholemeal breads and pastas, brown rice, plenty of vegetables and a little fruit for later meals.

Even simple canned baked beans, for example, are high in fibre and very low in fat. Like many canned foods, however, they are high in salt and salt reduced baked beans are preferable.

[3] Increase foods which help reduce cholesterol

Fish such as tuna is high in omega-3 fatty acids which help reduce blood cholesterol.

Linseed, pumpkin seed, soybean and canola oils are good sources of omega-3 and omega-6 fatty acids.

Bread varieties such as soy and linseed are therefore also a source of omega-3 oils. Soy protein also helps reduce cholesterol.

Garlic is also helpful in reducing cholesterol (Carper 2000) and is contained in many varieties of pasta sauce.

Highly coloured vegetables and fruits are rich in antioxidants which help reduce cholesterol absorption from food, good examples being tomatoes which are rich in lycopene, kidney beans, which are rich in phytosterols (sterols for short), and onions which are rich in the powerful antioxidant quercetin (Carper, 2000).

[4] Reduce sugar in the diet

Reducing sugar will help reduce triglyceride levels so reduce the amount of sugar in tea and coffee or, better still, use sugar substitutes.

If you must have cake and biscuits occasionally, eat only relatively plain cakes without icing and plain or dry biscuits, and dark chocolate with minimum fat and sugar content.

Avoid high-sugar confectionery as far as possible.

[5] Limit alcohol

The US Multiple Risk Factor Intervention Trial found that those of 11,000 middle-aged men who had two drinks a day for seven years had 22% fewer deaths from heart disease. Just one or two standard drinks a day, therefore, can be beneficial but avoid alcohol altogether if blood triglyceride levels are a concern (McGowan, 1998).

[6] Reduce salt in the diet

Too much salt raises blood pressure so hide the salt shaker and try to avoid packet and tinned soups, frozen and packaged meals, sauces high in salt, potato crisps and other salty snacks, salted nuts and canned tomato juice.

[7] Eat complex carbohydrates

Highly processed carbohydrates such as white sugar tend have a high *Glycemic Index* (GI) and increase blood sugar levels rapidly, thus being a risk to people with diabetes.

Generally, it is desirable for from 50 to 70% of our dietary calories to come from complex carbohydrates which tend to have low GI.

Lower GI foods include:

(a) Beans, peas and lentils.
(b) Nuts and seeds.
(c) Wholegrain breads, cereals, oats and muesli.
(d) Pasta and brown rice.
(e) Fruit and vegetables.

[8] Include a few nuts

Nuts are high in protein (and thence L-arginine), 'good' fats and many vitamins and minerals, including vitamin E, and one study found that people who eat them more than 5 times a week have 50% less heart disease than those who don't (Corder, 2007).

[9] Watch calories

Carefully count the calories in your diet to make sure you trim off any excess weight and then maintain a healthy weight.

An example diet

Table 17.1. Example diet, P = protein, C = carbs, F= fibre, Na = sodium.

Meal	Food	Cals	P gm	C gm	Fat gm	F gm	Na mg
Breakfast	3 wheat biscuits + skim milk	220	12	40	1.5	12	160
	200 ml breakfast juice	90	0.5	20	0	0.5	0
Morning	coffee + dash sugar/skim milk	20	0	4	0	0	30
Lunch	4 slices w/m bread + 50g tuna	365	26	52	6	8	640
	0.8L tea + sweetener/skim milk	40	1	9	0	0	50
Afternoon	2 slices bread + nut spread	200	16	30	8	4	320
	0.8L tea + sweetener/skim milk	40	1	9	0	0	50
Dinner	100 g tuna in spring water	80	20.5	0.5	0.5	0	135
	50 g mixed vegies	25	0.5	5	0	3	2
	50 g chips + dash chilli sauce	102	1.5	15	3	0.5	210
	coffee + dash sugar/skim milk	20	0	4	0	0	25
	one 150 g banana	100	2	22	0	3	0
Evening	120 ml glass red wine	90	2	21	0	0	25
	coffee + dash sugar/skim milk	20	0	4	0	0	30
	60 ml glass port wine	95	1	23	0	0	0
Bed	mug cocoa + skim milk	70	1	12	1	0	70
	35 g fruit cake	100	1.5	20	3	0.5	35
TOTAL		1,677	87	291	19.0	32	1,782
Percentage ot total calories			20.6	69.3	10.2		

Low fat diet plans for alternative days are shown in the Tables 17.1 and 17.2, the latter being vegetarian. Average daily calories is about 1650, about right for a physically inactive woman of over 55 and weighing 70 kg (Borushek, 2014). Individuals would, of course, adjust this two day diet plan to fit their own requirements. For example, a physically inactive man of over 55 and weighing 70 kg would require 2100 calories (Borushek, 2014).

Table 17.2. Example diet day 2 (vegetarian).

Meal	Food	Cals	P gm	C gm	Fat gm	F gm	Na mg
Breakfast	3 wheat biscuits + skim milk	220	12	40	1.5	12	160
	200 ml breakfast juice	90	0.5	20	0	0.5	0
Morning	coffee + dash sugar/skim milk	20	0	4	0	0	30
Lunch	pasta + mixed vegies + sauce	250	9	50	1.5	1	110
	0.8L tea + sweetener/skim milk	40	1	9	0	0	50
Afternoon	2 slices bread + nut spread	200	16	30	4	4	320
	0.8L tea + sweetener/skim milk	40	1	8	0	0	50
Dinner	200 g NAS baked beans	180	11	28	1	10	20
	50 g mixed vegies	25	0.5	5	0	3	2
	25 g chips + dash chilli sauce	51	0.7	7.5	1.5	0.25	105
	coffee + dash sugar/skim milk	20	0	4	0	0	30
	125 g peaches w/o syrup	100	0.5	24	0	3	0
Evening	120 ml glass red wine	90	2	21	0	0	25
	coffee + dash sugar/skim milk	20	0	4	0	0	30
	60 ml glass port wine	95	1	23	0	0	0
Bed	mug cocoa + skim milk	70	1	14	1	0	70
	35 g fruit cake	100	1.5	20	2.5	0.5	35
TOTAL		1,611	58	312	13.5	34	1,037
Percentage ot total calories			14.3	77.3	7.5		

Some of the measures taken to minimize fat and otherwise make the diets sounder included:

[1] Noting that saturated fats tend to be those which are solid at room temperature (Christensen, 2001), the sandwiches had for lunch in Table 17.1, and the bread + spread had with afternoon tea in both tables, are had without butter or margarine which are, of course, unnecessary.

[2] For the tuna dish, tuna in vegetable oil had once been used. Noting a report that some types of vegetable oil can lead to blindness in old age tuna in spring water was used instead.

[3] Wholemeal bread replaced biscuits and cake as snacks with afternoon tea.

For the author's height of almost 6'2" the minimum weight for a small frame is 73 kg, at his age requiring 2160 calories for a male, but another 300 calories is needed to sustain a moderate level of physical activity (Borushek, 2014). Without these additional calories, therefore, he lost weight gradually.

The primary goal of the diet was to satisfy the Kurzweil-Ornish-Pritikin 10% fat calories limit (Kurzweil, 1993) and this is very nearly achieved in Table 17.1, whilst fat intake is much less than 10% in Table 17.2.

Average protein intake is around the middle of the recommended range of 50 - 100 gm daily and also satisfies the long-standing rule that one gm of protein should be had for each kg of body weight.

Average carbohydrate intake is just above the range of 50 - 70% of total calories sometimes recommended, a situation difficult to avoid with an ultra-low fat diet.

Average fibre intake is within the 30 to 40 gm range recommended. In any case, with an ultra-low fat diet the fibre question is not quite so important as one is not counting on fibre to help reduce absorption of fat.

Sodium intake is well below the 2300 mg limit suggested by the NHMRC and the USFDA, and also below the American Heart Association 1500 mg limit.

Finally, note that the two glasses of wine had each evening might both be chilled dolce rosso in summer, and port wine in winter, rather than one of each as shown in Tables 17.1 and 17.2, or they might both be of red wine such as merlot.

Main features of the example diet

The main features of the example diet are:

[1] It aims to minimize fat and the average total fat content provides just under 9% of total calories, comfortably less than Kurzweil's 10% target (Kurzweil, 1993) to minimize cancer and heart disease risk.

[2] Fish is had every second day to provide protein and omega-3 fatty acids which help reduce blood cholesterol and are important for optimal brain function, for example being believed to be helpful in dealing with ADHD (Attention Deficit and Hyperactivity Disorder) in young children.

[3] Plenty of nutrient and antioxidant rich fruit and vegetables are had, tomato based pasta sauce also being a good source of the powerful antioxidant lycopene.

[4] Wheat flake biscuits and wholemeal bread and pasta help provide enough complex carbohydrate and fibre, and wholegrain pasta can be used to maximize the fibre content of the diet.

[5] Pasta sauce with garlic is used as garlic helps reduce blood cholesterol. Onion is also some help in this regard and is also had in the pasta sauce.

[6] Pots of tea are had after lunch and before dinner every day, tea being noted for its antioxidant properties. Green tea is a better source of antioxidants but was not used because many of its antioxidants are lost in drying.

[8] To help keep cholesterol concentrations in the blood down the diet involves total fluid well above the 2.5 litres minimum often recommended. In fact only about 75% of the pots of weak tea are actually consumed so that fluid consumption is actually circa 3.5 to 4 litres, about a litre less than shown in Tables 17.1 and 17.2.

Conclusions

The example diet passes most tests, in particular having calories from fat close to the minimal 10% figure suggested by Kurzweil (1993) to minimize cancer risk and normalize cholesterol levels.

$$2.5 \; L \; H_2O$$

177

Note, however, that it gives only enough calories for a basic level of physical activity for an inactive woman of over 55 and weighing 70 kg (Borushek, 2014). For even moderate levels of physical activity around 300 more calories are needed, and an example diet with about 500 more calories is given in the Appendix.

Notably, the only significant cooking effort involved is boiling pasta.

In contrast, many books on diet and health give reams of recipes involving countless ingredients which both the author and supermarket managers have never heard of and involve cooking for hours.

Note that, whilst the calorie total may need adjustment for different people with different activity levels, the diet objectives discussed in this chapter can be used as a basis for a sound diet for anyone.

Only two example diets were given in the foregoing chapter, but there many books full of healthy recipes are now available, for example *Low Fat Foods Fast* (Gold, 2002) and *The 10 Commandments of Losing Weight* (Normand, 2005). In addition, another example diet is given in the Appendix.

Finally, note that "scientific studies suggest that about 30 percent of all cancer deaths are associated with poor dietary and nutrition practices" (Ko et. al., 2008).

Chapter 18

DIETARY SUPPLEMENT PLAN

> the Pracon Study, commissioned by the Council for Responsible Nutrition,
> estimated that $8.7 billion could be saved on
> five major diseases if Americans consumed optimal levels
> of the antioxidants vitamin C, vitamin E, and beta-carotene.
> Prof. HG Preuss MD in the foreword to
> *The Real Vitamin & Mineral Book*, Liebermann & Bruning (1997).

Some important diet supplements

As early chapters indicate, small quantities of vitamins and other key nutrients such as omega-3 oils can play a crucial role in reducing the risks of heart disease and cancer.

In the Appendix it is shown that the example diet of the preceding chapter is a little short on vitamin E. It is also a little low on zinc, a mineral important for good prostate gland function. Absorption of dietary zinc can be severely reduced by excessive alcohol consumption and this perhaps is, in part at least, and explanation for an increasing incidence of prostate problems and cancer.

For such reasons dietary supplements are worthwhile for most, if not all, people. Some of the most important supplements are:

{1} **Fish oil.** Fish oil in the diet has been proved to reduce incidence of heart attacks by about 30% (Carper 2000) and omega-3 fish oils may help reduce arterial plaques.

[2] **Garlic oil.** Fish oil increases LDL slightly but garlic offsets this problem and also helps shrink arterial plaques, thus reducing incidence of fatal heart attacks by up to 66% (Carper 2000).

[3] Niacin

Niacin, or the nicotinic acid form of vitamin B3, assists fat metabolism and has been shown to reduce cholesterol levels and is widely used in the USA for this purpose (Kowalski, 1987; McGowan, 1998), but requires dosages of from 2 - 3 grams daily to be effective.

As little as 50 - 100 mg can cause facial and upper body 'flushing' symptoms and headaches in some people, however, but sustained release formulations are available which reduce this problem (Kowalski, 2006) though Cooper (1996) notes that there is some risk of liver damage with continued use of these.

A relatively new alternative natural supplement for lowering cholesterol levels is Policosanol which Kowalski (2006) suggests requires further proof of its effectiveness.

[4] Folate

Heber in his book *Natural Remedies for a Healthy Heart* takes the view that homocysteine is a greater villain than cholesterol in the cardiovascular story and notes that levels of this are high in 42% of cerebrovascular, 30% of cardiovascular and 28% of peripheral vascular disease patients. Indeed, elevated homocysteine levels triple the risk of heart attack or stroke.

Folate, also known as folic acid and vitamin B9, helps reduce homocysteine levels.

Another benefit of folate was reported in a 2005 paper in the *British Medical Journal.* It reported research that found that a high folate intake helped negate the increased risk of breast cancer in women who had high levels of alcohol consumption.

[5] Antioxidants

Antioxidant Vitamins A, C and E are important because water soluble C soaks up potentially mutagenic free radicals within the cell and fat-soluble A and E soak them up in the cell membrane. Together they therefore increase immunity to cancer and other diseases.

Vitamin C also helps maintain healthy blood vessel walls whilst vitamin E can reduce heart attack risk by up to 75% in people with minor arterial disease. The Cambridge Heart Antioxidant Study found that after a first heart attack 400 IU of vitamin E almost halved risk of a second.

Vitamin E can reduce moderate-sized arterial plaques but not major ones, and then only before arteries have become fibrotic and permanently hardened. As always, therefore, prevention is better than cure, and antioxidants are important in this regard.

18. Dietary Supplement Plan

A 1977 book by Dr Atkins on his low carbohydrate diet notes the promise of vitamin A in dealing with cancer and the Dutch-government-approved Moerman anti-cancer therapy uses megadoses of vitamins A, C and E, including an almost toxic dose of vitamin A. It is synthetic derivatives of vitamin A (retinoids), however, that show more promise in inhibiting and perhaps regressing cancer (Mohr, 2012b, 2013).

Ongoing research is exploring the belief that selenium and vitamin E taken together can reduce the incidence of some cancers by as much as a whopping 50%.

CoQ10 is an antioxidant made by the body which is synergistic with vitamins C and E and it also reduces oxidation of cholesterol in blood vessel walls. CoQ10 supplementation is widely used for patients who have suffered heart failure because it reduces shortness of breath and thence hospitalizations. The author found magnesium + CoQ10 powder a convenient way of taking CoQ10.

[6] Minerals
Magnesium in water supplies has been found to reduce heart attack rates because it reduces arrhythmia which makes heart attacks more likely to be fatal. Magnesium has also been found to halve cardiovascular complications in high-risk patients, reduce angina, and has even been injected to increase survival rates from heart attack.

Magnesium can also reduce, if not prevent, variant angina.

Phosphorus as phosphate assists in energy metabolism and is a powerful antioxidant.

Several other minerals are important for proper health, for example iron to prevent iron deficiency anemia, calcium to prevent osteoporosis, and zinc to help prevent and treat benign prostate hypertrophy (BPH), a disorder very common in older men.

[7] Aspirin
Taking half to one aspirin a day is widely recommended as aspirin reduces blood vessel inflammation and thins the blood, and thus reduces the risk of congestive stroke. It may, however, increase the severity of a haemorraghic stroke.

Note in passing that hot climates also increase the risk of haemorraghic stroke. To state the obvious, this suggests that people susceptible to or with a history of stroke should avoid overexertion, especially in hot weather.

Short and medium term supplementation

Table 18.1 shows the short-term and medium-term dietary supplementation used by the author in conjunction diet of Chapter 17.

Table 18.1. Diet supplementation plan. Note that older women should also take additional calcium supplements + vitamin D daily.

Supplement	Short-term (6 months)	Medium term (1 - 2 years)
Fish oil (omega-3) capsule, 1g	3 daily	1 daily
Garlic oil capsule, 3 g	1 daily	1 daily
0.5 gm L-arginine	3 daily	
Lysine	As per Table 3.2	
100 mg niacin	3-6 daily	
Policosanal, 5 or 10 mg	1 daily for 50 days	
500 mcg folid acid + 500 mcg B12 + 250 mg calcium	daily for 3 months	
Vitamin A, 5000 IU	1 daily	
Vitamin C, 500 mg	1 daily	1 daily
Vitamin E, 400 IU	1 daily	1 weekly
Magnesium, 325 mg	2 daily	2 daily
Multivitamin incl. A, B1 - B6, B12, D3, E betacarotene, calcium, iron, potassium, selenium & zinc	1 daily	1 daily
Aspirin	2 x ½ daily	½ daily
Lecithin & linseeds with meals	7.5 gm of each twice daily	7.5 gm of each daily

This diet supplementation program involves:

[1] To help maintain good blood cholesterol levels and reduce risk of heart attack fish oil (30% omega-3) and garlic oil capsules are taken.

[2] Moderate dosage L-arginine is taken for 6 months to promote NO production and thence endothelial relaxation, whilst lysine is taken according to Table 3.2.

[3] High-dose niacin may improve cholesterol levels substantially but without prescription is only available in Australia in 100 mg tablets of which a bottle of 100 might only last just over 3 days at the level of 3 grams/day dosage recommended by Kowalski (1987).

As an alternative, therefore:

(a) A modest dose of three to six 100 mg niacin tablets are taken daily to help reduce cholesterol levels.

(b) Policosanol is also used as a short-term supplement to improve serum cholesterol levels, taking 5 mg and 10 mg Policosanol tablets alternately for 40 days, followed by 5 mg tablets for a further 10 days. This gave nearly the 8-week period of dosage for which good results had been obtained during trials with 31,000 people over periods of 2 - 5 years.

[3] In months 1 - 3 of the program one tablet with 500 mcg of folic acid, 500 mcg of vitamin B12 and 250 mg of calcium is taken daily. This gives slightly more than the 400 mcg of folate required daily to normalize homocysteine levels in three months.

[4] Vitamins A, C, E are also taken, but only in moderation. The main aim of the present book is that of increased health and immunity, not cure, though reversal of vascular disease is intended, so that only modest vitamin A supplementation is had.

[5] Magnesium is taken daily as this assists vascular expansion and thus helps prevent variant or stress angina. Magnesium as Epsom Salts (hydrated magnesium sulphate) is used to alleviate constipation and thus magnesium supplements taken regularly will help clear the bowels more rapidly, helping weight loss or preventing weight gain.

[8] To make sure nothing was missing in the way of key vitamins and minerals comprehensive multivitamin and mineral tablets are included.

[9] Aspirin has been found to reduce heart attacks by 44% but must be taken daily to be effective. It also reduces risk of stroke and has been found to reduce colon cancer by 44% in one study.

[10] Lecithin and linseeds daily as noted in Chapters 2 and 3.

Note that, as shown in Table 3.2, dosages of C, E, lysine, L-arginine, niacin and magnesium can be adjusted according to whether one suffers 'effort angina' or 'stress /variant angina'.

The plan should give 'feeling better' results in weeks, if not days, but to normalize cholesterol levels some people might find it necessary to have high-dose niacin or medication and to extend the initial 6-month plan to 12 months or more.

Comments

Some of the supplements included in the program of Table 18.1 are intended as 'catch up' measures, not as permanent. Folic acid supplementation to normalize homocysteine levels, for example, is only necessary for a few months and in the longer term one should be able to obtain sufficient quantities of most nutrients from food.

In developing a supplement program the startling results claimed for lecithin and noted in Chapter 2 sprang to attention. If one believed these, lecithin may be beneficial for a wide variety of complaints including atherosclerotic heart disease, peripheral vascular disease, varicose veins, high and low BP, high cholesterol, arthritis, bursitis, phlebitis, glaucoma, and Alzheimer's and Parkinson's diseases (Murray, 1977; Fischer, 1993).

Just how lecithin might be so beneficial was clear, that is:

(a) By way of its emulsifying action on blood fats.

(b) Because of its role in facilitating passage of cholesterol through cell membranes.

(c) Through its reverse cholesterol transport role as a key component of HDL.

It is through these actions that lecithin is the crucial ingredient in the famous Dr Rinse Formula discussed in Chapter 2, bonemeal only being required to deal with osteoporosis, and omega-rich seed oils to provide a secondary and supportive role to that of lecithin.

Note that one capusule of bioactivated resveratrol is equivalent to 1000 glasses of red wine and therefore well worth taking occasionally.

For many people prescribed medications for high BP or to normalize cholesterol might be required. Again, however, every effort should be made to make these a short-term option by improving diet and exercise regimes and using the natural supplements such as niacin, L-arginine and L-lysine discussed in Chapters 12 and 13.

Finally, note that older women should take calcium + D supplements daily, while older men should take zinc and 'prostate formula' tablets including saw palmetto, nettle extract and pygeum. Pomegranate juice is also beneficial, its antioxidant punicalagins having been found most effective in helping cure prostate cancer. For those exercising to rebuild spent muscle protein powders are also worthwhile.

Chapter 19

EXERCISE AND RELAXATION

> *In fact, exercise is one of the most important single factors
> contributing to cardiovascular health.*
> Dr Robert Superko, *Before the Heart Attacks* (2004).

Introduction

A comprehensive health plan should involve:

[1] A carefully analyzed diet

The first step in calculating daily calorie intake is the most important as this can be the major step in losing weight, if necessary. Then, of course, one should eliminate the 'bad things' like saturated fat as far as possible, and substitute healthy things like fish and vegetables. Finally, it is important to analyze the diet, as in Chapter 17, to check intake of protein, carbohydrates, fat and salt.

[2] An ongoing program of dietary supplements

Most doctors recommend at least a multivitamin tablet and, if you are older, half an aspirin daily to cut risk of heart attack and stroke.

But to minimize aging and risk of heart disease and cancer synergistic selenium and vitamins C and E should be considered, along with omega-3 oils by way of fish oil capsules or seed oils.

For those concerned with cholesterol levels such supplements as niacin, Policosanol and lecithin should be considered. Just as important, folate and B12 should be taken for a few months to normalize homocysteine levels. Those concerned with prostate health should take zinc whilst lecithin may be beneficial for a wide range of issues.

[3] A comprehensive exercise program

A comprehensive exercise program should include walking, calisthenics, jogging (however slow), exercise bike sessions and at least a few weight exercises daily, no matter how light the weights, the number of reps being more important for heart health.

Household and garden chores may provide additional exercise.

19. Exercise and Relaxation

[4] Stress reduction and relaxation

It is widely believed that stress is just about as important a factor in heart problems as any other. Some efforts at stress reduction, therefore, are well worthwhile. At the simplest level these may just involve taking things that one tends to rush or find stressful a little slower.

Periods of 'relaxation therapy' should also be considered, ranging from, for example, simply sitting back and listening to relaxing music to meditation techniques and yoga.

Example exercise program - stage 1

For those of us that have neglected exercise by and large, it is prudent to build up exercise programs gradually. For those with serious health problems it is downright necessary.

By way of example only, my initial exercise program to improve cardiovascular health progressed as follows:

[1] First week

As much walking as possible and averaging more than an hour a day.

[2] Running

After the first week a run around small lake in a large park nearby whenever possible. Never having been a long distance runner I broke this into four short stretches. The first was up a fairly steep embankment and this got his heart rate near the top of the target range. The rest of the circuit was fairly undulating and made for good exercise and the remaining three stretches of the circuit around the lake got heart rate above the middle of the target heart rate range.

Between these four running stretches toe touches, pushups and other calisthenics exercises were done. This 'circuit around the lake plus calisthenics' was then repeated for a second time. After a few weeks I increased to three repetitions of this lake circuit drill.

[3] Indoor exercises

These comprised 'knees up running on the spot' followed by pushups, toe touches, squats and various calisthenics such as twists of the waist and neck and twirls of the arms.

Finally, to help keep my back supple I also touched my toes (as nearly as I could easily) 20 times before having my daily shower.

These indoor drills I did daily.

[4] Resistance work

After a few months I bought a barbell and some modest weights with a total of only 23 kg (51 lb).

After a few experiments I settled on doing a set which averaged out at about 15 reps of above head lifts, 15 reps of barbell curls and 15 reps of barbell squats. This I found got my heart rate up near the top of the target range and thus served as both an aerobic and a resistance drill.

Barbell squats exercise the largest muscle groups and I found doing 15 squats hard enough without any weights and that 20 - 30 kilos or so of extra weight did not make them much harder than they already were.

I did this set of reps an average of about three or four times a week, increasing the weight and decreasing the number of reps after three weeks as in the example program given in Chapter 7 in the section *Building up strength*.

A word of caution. Note that I had already been doing what was, for me, a fairly solid exercise effort for four months before I began using these quite modest weights. Readers should take great care to test themselves with the smallest possible weights to get an idea of what sort of weights to begin a weight program with.

Note that, in people who have had a previous heart attack, the probability of another attack is found to be primarily determined by their *physical capacity*. Thus it has been found that heart rates after measured exercise on a treadmill are sometimes a better indication of heart health than ECG tests.

Example exercise program - stage 2

The main improvement was that I merged the short stages of my run routine into a continuous run, the duration of which I gradually increased from 5 minutes to 30 minutes, a lifetime record! This I did once a week.

I also got an exercise bike and used this for a few minutes after my weights exercises.

Finally, I tried to do a two-hour walk sometimes as my heart, which had given me occasional symptoms for 30 years, had often given regular very slight discomfort after 30 minutes walking.

Example exercise program - stage 3

Towards the end of my occasional long walks of nearly two hours, however, I author found that I was experiencing very mild angina pectoris. It was clear that an improved exercise routine was needed. To this end, therefore, the following improvements were made:

(1) An improved 'gym drill' daily involving:
(a) A lighter weight on the bar with a larger number of reps, still doing brackets of above head lifts, curls and squats consecutively without a break. This took about two minutes.

The point here is that larger numbers of reps (with lesser weights) gives a combination of endurance and strength which is better for heart health (Cooke & Zimmer, 2002).
(b) Five minutes on the exercise bike with a minute at 75% maximum effort and the last minute at top effort. (b) was done straight after (a) without a break.

(2) The now 30 minute non-stop run was done twice a week.

(3) For flexibility a daily calisthenics routine of pushups and half a dozen other movements was done, followed by a minute or two running on the spot with 'knees up' as much as possible.

In addition, 20 'toe touches' were still done before daily before showering to keep the back supple.

(4) At least half an hour's walking was done every day.

(5) An additional walk of about an hour or so was done on most days, extending this to somewhere near two hours once or twice a week.

The resulting weekly program is summarized in Table 19.1.
Here walking is assumed to be at around a modest 3.5 miles per hour, consuming only 5 calories per minute, whereas the other exercises consume calories at a much greater rate.

The number of minutes of each exercise undertaken for each day of the week is recorded in spreadsheet, allowing the total number of calories for the day to be calculated in the last column as

+B4*B2+C4*C2+D4*D2+E4*E2

for Sunday, this calculation being 'dragged' to the cells below it in the final column.

Table 19.1. Spreadsheet exercise record showing minutes per day of each type of exercise undertaken.

Exercise:	Walk	Aerobic	Run	Gym	Total
Cals/min	5	11	8	11	calories
Day	(B)	(C)	(D)	(E)	
Sun	60	3	30	7	650
Mon	60	3	0	7	410
Tue	60	3	0	7	410
Wed	60	3	0	7	410
Thur	60	3	30	7	650
Fri	60	3	0	7	410
Sat	60	3	0	7	410
Total	420	21	60	49	3,350

The number of calories that need to be consumed to work off a pound in weight (450 gm) for the 'average' person is about 3,500 calories and the calorie total for the week in Table 19.1 is close to this. Remembering that one gm of fat equates to 9 calories but one gm of protein to only 4 calories, it is clear that when we do lose weight through exercise most of it is fat, otherwise we would lose weight far more rapidly.

Calorie requirements

One's calorie requirements can be calculated using the Harris-Benedict equations for *basal metabolic rate* or BMR:

Men:

BMR = 66 + 13.7 X kg weight + 5 X cm height - 6.8 X years age

Women:

BMR = 655 + 9.6 X kg weight + 1.8 X cm height - 4.7 X years age

For a man 45 years old, 179 cm tall, and weighing 75 kg
   BMR = 66 + 13.7 X 75 + 5 X 179 - 6.8 X 45 = 1682 calories

For a woman 45 years old, 169 cm tall, and weighing 60 kg
   BMR = 655 + 9.6 X 60 + 1.8 X 169 - 4.7 X 45 = 1324 calories

These are the calories required to lie in bed and do nothing. For various rates of activity these results should be multiplied by the following factors:

1.2 for sedentary, i.e., desk job and little or no exercise

1.375 for a little active, i.e., light exercise 1 to 3 days/week

1.55 for moderately active, i.e., moderate exercise 3 to 5 days/week

1.725 for very active, i.e., hard exercise 6 to 7 days/week

1.9 for super active, i.e., hard physical job + hard exercise daily

Then for the example man and woman above we obtain for moderate activity:

Man: 1682 X 1.55 = 2607 calories

Woman: 1324 X 1.55 = 2051 calories

For a man and woman with the same specifications the results obtained in Chapter 6 were respectively 2650 and 1850 calories, so the present BMR calculations give a result about 10% higher in the woman's case.

Extra calories for exercise

When additional exercise is done more calories are needed to provide the energy for it. One should be at pains to ensure that these extra calories are not from convenient but unhealthy fat-laden snack foods or alcohol. An example might be having 3 litres of full strength beer and 200 gm of potato crisps, yielding around 2200 calories, more than the average daily total for the example diets of Chapter 17.

The bad news is that 33% of this is fat, far above the desirable lower limit of 10%. Worse still, if this binge is had after having one's dinner and thus most of a normal day's food, then the result is almost two day's worth of food in one and thus a considerable overnight boost to blood cholesterol levels.

A recent study showed that just one unhealthy meal can reduce the body's defences against heart attack and stroke. 14 healthy adults aged 18 to 40 were given identical meals one month apart, except that one had one gram of saturated fat per kg of body weight and the other the same amount of polyunsaturated fat (safflower oil). The single meal high in saturated fat increased inflammation in the arteries and reduced their ability to expand (SJ Nicholls et al., *J Amer Coll Cardiol*, 48 (2006) 715-720).

The best practice, therefore, is to make up for a calorie shortfall over a few days by simply increasing serving sizes or by adding small amounts of snacks such as raw baby carrots, nuts, dried fruit, muesli bars or whole-grain biscuits.

Here even a little dark chocolate is permissible. Chocolate is high in both fat and sugar but, fortunately, much of the fat in dark chocolate is from cocoa fat which is not as harmful as animal fat.

Cocoa also contains antioxidant polyphenols similar to those in fruit and vegetables. These reduce the harmful oxidation of cholesterol and protect nitric oxide (NO.) In addition, some of the polyphenols in chocolate increase NO production (more importantly, so does exercise). Thus occasional small amounts of chocolate, particularly dark chocolate, are actually beneficial, even to heart patients (Cooke & Zimmer, 2002).

Alcohol in moderation will provide extra calories and, until recently, in Australia health authorities recommended four standard drinks a day as OK for men, and two for women. Indeed, as discussed in Chapter 6, a couple of glasses of red wine a day almost halves risk of heart attack.

Summary

Your own exercise program might be very different from that of the author and given herein but it should follow the principles of:

(a) Involving a *variety* of activities such as calisthenics, walking both short and long distances, cycling (perhaps on an exercise bike), jogging, and using modest weights with a substantial number of reps.

Longer walks, for example, might be achieved by playing golf, though surely long, brisk and continuous walks must be better exercise and a good deal less stressful than golf can often be.

(b) Slowly building up such activities as walking, jogging and resistance training over months and years, making sure that some of your exercise program gets you well into your target heart rate range, preferably two or three or more times every day.

Relaxation

Having purchased a 'strap on' electronic blood pressure monitor the author was surprised to note that straight after his 30 minute run or fairly hectic nonstop gym drill his BP was only about 135/85, not much higher as he had expected. After one period of dietary and exercise lapse, on the other hand, he had had BP readings of up to 200/120 when mentally stressed.

The message was clear, namely that:

(a) 'Relaxing' in the traditional fashion by, for example, having booze to celebrate Christmas and New Year, can do more harm than good and even be life threatening if you are only halfway fragile.

(b) Genuine relaxation is important and healthy.

The following are just a few examples of the many ways in which we can try and relax a little better:

[1] Plenty of sleep.

This may simply involve not getting up early unless strictly necessary. BP is higher in the morning and I recall only too well a visiting nurse dragging my very fragile father out of bed soon after 9 AM one morning and him having a stroke and not living long after it. This sort of lunacy goes on in hospitals and nursing homes, of course, taking little notice of the fact that our BP tends to be highest in the mornings, a phenomenon known as 'morning surge' (Kowalski, 2006).

About eight hours sleep is the amount generally recommended but this might involve fewer hours of 'quality sleep.' It is therefore best to often have an extra hour or two in bed make sure you have enough truly good quality sleep each week.

Indeed, a recent study found that children aged from 3 to 18 were at greater risk of being overweight if they didn't get enough sleep (E Snell et al., *Child Dev.* vol. 78). Presumably, the reason for this otherwise apparently contradictory finding is that those who stayed up late or arose early were prone to indulge in additional snacks, whereas those who got up just in the nick of time to get to school might well be forced to have a light breakfast if any at all.

[2] Yoga and meditation techniques. Some of these were briefly discussed in Chapter 9.

[3] An occasional hot bath. This is not only relaxing, but presumably is good for one's circulation too.

[4] Turn the TV off and listen to some quiet classical, jazz or relaxation music each evening.

[5] Have a quiet couple of hours each evening having a slow couple of glasses of red wine or other favourite nonalcoholic drink.

[6] Watch TV in bed if you want to see the end of some TV show that runs past your usual bed time.

[7] Take longer walks in relaxing surroundings such as through parks or by the beach.

[8] Shopping, especially window-shopping, can also be a relaxing pastime while also giving you a little exercise.

[9] Spend the odd hour playing a PC (or Playstation etc.) game, for example one of the many excellent chess programs available.

[10] Spend a while each day quietly reading newspapers, magazines or books. Reading in bed is especially relaxing, perhaps with some quite background music playing on your radio alarm.

[11] Make sure you keep up one or two hobbies to help pass spare time. These might include useful activities like knitting and sewing or other useful and healthy activities like gardening.

[12] Make sure you have regular social contacts, for example at one of the many types of clubs and societies around these days. In these, no doubt, you will make new friends and, in turn, find new ways to fill in your spare time with relaxing activities.

Conclusion

Used only to obligatory walking for errands, my exercise program started with minimal calisthenics while something was cooking and, over years, built up to jogging for longer than I ever had before and beginning to use weights sensibly. That is, with lower weights and larger numbers of repetitions, with the aim of better endurance and heart health, being prepared to wait months before increasing the weights slightly, when I found the same number of reps possible straight away.

As for relaxation, this may be more a question of eliminating activities that are not really relaxing and retaining or reviving others that are. By way of example, the following are not really particularly relaxing or sensible:

(a) Moping around pubs or clubs with a drink in your hand.

(b) Doing likewise at parties or other functions.

(c) Stewing over the score in some team ball game while holding a drink in your hand. It might make more sense these days if they announced the scores at the outset and let the highly paid sports performers act out the game accordingly, complete with the ludicrous operatic histrionics both they and some of the more deranged and/or intoxicated spectators increasingly indulge in now.

Sitting in a comfortable armchair at home slowly drinking a glass of port is more like it if you really want to relax. Now that we all know that alcohol might only be of benefit in medicinal doses, and then only if you are middle aged or older, this indeed seems the only appropriate way to drink it. The result will immediately be an improved, more relaxing lifestyle, and also better health in the long term.

Bottom line

Note that only 9-12% of the high heart risk middle-aged men with total cholesterol levels above 240 mg/dl actually have symptoms of cardiovascular disease as a direct result.

The bottom line is that you should develop a healthy diet and exercise plan which:

(a) Eliminates or minimizes all the unhealthy things like smoking, alcohol, salt, sugar, fat, stress and slothfulness.

(b) Includes as many as possible of the healthy things like fruit and vegetables, whole grains, antioxidants and other nutrients.

(c) Involves aerobic and strength building exercises.

(d) Involves stress reduction and relaxation.

(e) Ensures that you have acceptable cholesterol, homocysteine, blood pressure, weight and body fat levels.

Finally, there is much DIY emphasis in the present book but if you have even halfway serious health problems, however, do not hesitate to seek professional advice.

Chapter 20

8-WEEK PROGRAM
TO REDUCE BP & CHOLESTEROL

> In no uncertain terms, you are as young as your arteries.
> Having high blood pressure can make a person's Real Age
> more than twenty-five years older than having low blood pressure.
> Michael Roizen, *Real Age, Are You as Young as You Can Be?* (2001).

An 8-week program

In the present chapter the diet of Tables 17.1 and 17.2 is tightened slightly and exercise is increased to lose a little weight and decrease cholesterol levels and reduce blood pressure. In line with Kowalski's *8-Week Cholesterol Cure*, the program is for 8-weeks (Kowalski, 1987). Then, as shown in Table 16.2, the higher levels of exercise of Kurweil's low fat diet program dramatically improve cholesterol levels (Kurzweil, 1993).

The purpose of this is not to kill unfit or older people who are advised to stick to exercises more of the 'rehab' type, but to target the high risk group for heart disease, namely middle aged men who have 'let themselves go' with poor diet and lack of exercise since their early 20s, if not their teens, and thence 'gone to pot' and developed a 'pot belly'.

Many women, of course, have the same problem. Not only that, many men have seemingly solid exercise routines but still find themselves on the heart surgeon's operating table and wonder why (Kowalski, 1987). This may be because they concentrate on just one form of relatively monotonous exercise such as walking, golf or slow jogging and do little to improve their diet.

The 8-week program diet

The changes to the diet of Tables 17.1 and 17.2 are:

(1) A tablespoon of heart healthy olive or canola oil (both of which are monounsaturated) was often added to dinner.

(2) No milk was had with the 2 pots of tea had per day. This is because a recent small German study of 16 healthy post-menopausal women (European Heart Journal, 2006) showed that just drinking black tea on only three occasions significantly improved *Flow Mediated Dilation* (FMD) of their arteries for weeks afterwards, but only if no milk was had with the tea. It was concluded that the caseins in skim milk interfered with the antioxidant action of the flavonoids in the tea which help prevent heart disease and cancer. Thus the many people who have no sugar with their tea in a usually token and vain effort at calorie and weight trimming have it wrong. Better to have a little raw sugar in the tea for flavour than to have any kind of milk and it is easy to compensate for the few calories involved elsewhere if need be.

(3) As an alternative to the red wine had in the evening dark grape juice is often had which is also rich in procyanidins and has up to 50% of the antioxidant action of red wine (Corder, 2007).

(4) To help add muscle while burning up fat 25gm Testosteroid powder, a testofen enhanced protein formula, was taken mixed with water daily. Testofen improves testosterone balance and the formula also contains 18 essential amino acids, including methionine which improves muscle function.

Upping the exercise

One expert recommends exercise as the best means of tackling heart disease (Kiat 2002). Another writer on the subject points out that the best way to reduce blood triglyceride levels is exercise and the sooner the better (Murray 1977). Thus if you have celebrated a little at Christmas, for example, the best way to make sure your TG levels are OK is to work them down with exercise ASAP before conversion to VLDL, LDL and thence atheroma takes place.

In one study four sedentary days were followed by running 3-4 miles in circa 40 minutes on four successive afternoons, after which average TG levels fell from 235 to 173, 136, 119, and 104. Then after 3-7 days of sedentary recovery TG levels returned to their baseline levels Murray (1977).

A report on a study published in the *International Journal of Obesity* in 2007 found that 20 minutes of exercise of variable intensities was more effective than 40 minutes of steady-state exercise in burning off body fat and increasing aerobic fitness (*The Weekend Australian* 27-28 Jan. 2007).

Table 20.1. Circuit training drill.

Part	Exercise	Equipment	Reps
1	cheat overhead press	barbell (25 kg)	40
	cheat curl	barbell	30
	upright row	barbell	30
	barbell bent over row	barbell	40
	barbell squat and lift	barbell	30
2	leg extension (seated)	ankle weights (4.5 kg)	2 X 50
	1 arm dumbbell lateral fly *	dumbbell (7.5 kg)	2 X 30
	1 arm bench press *	dumbbell	2 X 30
	2 arm dumbbell back swing *	dumbbell	20
	2 arm dumbbell forward swing *	dumbbell	30
	trunk curl (lying on floor)	none	25
	twisting trunk curl (" ")	none	25
	* = reclining		
3	1 arm dumbbell press	dumbbell (7 kg)	2 X 30
	1 arm dumbbell lateral swing	dumbbell	2 X 30
	weighted side bend (both sides)	2 dumbbells	50
	1 arm curl	dumbbell	2 X 30
	1 arm supported dumbbell bent over row	dumbbell	2 X 30
	triceps extension	dumbbell	30
4	bike	exercise bike	5 min

Such a variable exercise intensity is provided by the circuit training routine shown in Table 20.1. Some of the terms used to describe the exercises are similar to those used conventionally in the fitness industry (Sudy, 1991). For those not familiar with some of them it is hoped they are nevertheless reasonably self-evident.

In any event a couple of the exercises are original inventions of the mine and, given a barbell and a dumbbell or two, readers will be able to do likewise. They should take special care, however, to use modest weights in line with their physical condition at the outset.

Moving from one element to the next with as little delay as possible the entire drill should take about half an hour.

During my 8-week special effort I repeated the entire drill with only a minute or two break before doing so. This provided me with a really solid workout for almost the first time. I did this 'double drill' every day, reducing my run to once a week.

I also did at least half an hour's walking a day, and usually an hour, also keeping up a lunch time calisthenics and running on the spot routine every day, doing my 30 minute run only weekly because the daily one hour gym effort rarely left either time or energy for it.

After only a couple of weeks the results were excellent, upper body circulation and muscle condition improving considerably.

Long term exercise plan

After I had completed my 8-week program of exercise and diet I did the exercise routine of Table 20.1 only once in a session, taking about half an hour, and then only a couple of times a week.

Sometimes, when I couldn't find time for the full half hour drill, just the first barbell part and the fourth bike part of Table 20.1 were done, leaving the two dumbbell parts until the evening or the next day.

In place of the daily gym drill I got a road bike and used this and an exercise bike for a total of half an hour or more daily.

I also kept up a lunch time calisthenics routine of two minutes followed by on the spot running, increasing the latter to four minutes with about half of this in sprint or 'knees up mode.'

Noting that my metabolic or at rest rate of energy consumption was about 1.25 calories per minute (Borushek, 2014) I estimated that my exercise efforts involved the following *additional* energy requirements per minute:

Gym drill: + 10 calories/minute.
Calisthenics + 'sprints' routine: + 10 calories/minute.
Road or exercise bike: + 6 calories/minute.
Jogging: + 7 calories/minute.
Walking: + 4 calories/minute.
Lawn mowing or housework like vacuuming: + 3 calories/minute.

Then, for example, on a day when the exercise efforts are lunchtime calisthenics (6 minutes), the half hour gym drill, half an hour on a bike and an hour's walking, exercise calorie consumption can be calculated as

$$6 \times 10 + 30 \times 10 + 30 \times 6 + 60 \times 4 = 780 \text{ calories}$$

This is the equivalent of about three hours walking, an amount of exercise sure to increase one's fitness. Indeed, bearing in mind that variable exercise intensity is best at burning up fat and at developing real fitness this varied exercise program was far better than the walking that had been relied upon mostly for exercise in the past.

Day in, day out, one should do at least something like 300 to 400 calories of 'dedicated' exercise effort. It is also a good idea to try to increase this to nearer 700 calories a day for 2 to 4 weeks a year to achieve a better level of fitness.

Note in passing that the additional calorie values used here are approximately the same as the widely used Metabolic Equivalent or MET values (Luckman & Sorenson, 1980; Kowalski, 2006).

An initial 40-day program

Table 20.2 shows the BP readings I obtained during a 40 day program in 2005 when my efforts at tackling heart disease were in their early stages (Mohr, 2012b; Mohr, 2013).

Here the results are given for eight five-day periods.

During my 40-day 'crash program' my weight dropped to about 150 pounds or 67 kg, considerably lower than I had originally aimed for. Taking my height to be 6 ft 1 inch (it is actually somewhere between 6'1" and 6'2") my Body Mass Index (BMI) was

$$(\text{weight in kg})/(\text{height in metres})^2 = 19.4$$

Less than 18 or 19 would be underweight (Borushek, 2014; Kowalksi, 2006) so this result showed that I had indeed removed as much fat as possible, leaving only a pound or two of 'pinchable' waistline fat and giving the best chance of minimizing blood cholesterol and regressing atherosclerosis.

Table 20.2. Average BP readings during eight consecutive 5-day periods.

Period	Systolic	Diastolic
1	158	93
2	139	78
3	131	75
4	141	76
5	142	74
6	139	75
7	138	85
8	136	89

Finally, after the 40-day program and the years of slowly developing exercise routines before it, my resting pulse rate (RPR) was usually about 60 and sometimes well below that, a result I could not recall achieving at any other stage of life.

My heart symptoms that I had had quite often in previous years began to disappear, for example the heart region or shoulder pain that I had experienced with walks of half an hour at one stage, and about two hours at another stage, were almost completely gone.

I still, however, experienced unpredictable heart pains at times of stress, often while doing seemingly trivial manual things around the house, this being variant (stress) angina (not effort angina), and for this I take magnesium daily with excellent results.

I am now convinced, however, that for those of us inclined to impatience, such activities working at pace at a desk, cooking, or dish washing, are unhealthy because we feel stressed so that adrenalin will contract our blood vessels.

There is not, however, enough physical effort to get the heart pumping harder and really open up blood vessels as there is with exercise which raises the heart rate substantially, over time strengthening the heart, and reducing blood pressure and cholesterol levels.

The 8-week program

Table 20.3 shows the results I obtained during an 8-week 'refresher' program in early 2015 to reduce BP, having for a few months let my diet slip during the very stressful effort of completing my memoirs which was a somewhat melancholy task to say the least. The table also shows the data for the week '0' before the 8-week program began.

Table 20.3. Results for 8-week program.

Week	Exercise Cals/day	Diet	Stress	Average BP Systolic	Diastolic	Average RPR
0	800	X	X	132	64	80
1	800	OK	OK	122	60	69
2	700	OK	OK	116	61	60
3	650	OK	OK	102	53	61
4	600	OK	OK	111	60	62
5	700	OK	OK	115	60	63
6	650	OK	OK	106	56	63
7	550	OK	OK	109	63	60
8	700	OK	OK	109	58	63

The first week alone considerably improved BP and pulse rate, further improvement being obtained in following weeks until BP and RPR were relatively low.

Not for the first time, a few months of hectic work with dietary lapses had resulted in stasis dermatitis on an ankle but this had almost disappeared after only four weeks of the 8-week program and I was feeling a good deal healthier overall with my diet back on track and remained determined to keep it that way.

A few notes on BP readings

The importance of blood pressure needs little emphasis and the WHO estimated recently that 11 per cent of all significant disease in developed countries is caused by high BP alone.

For reference purposes BP readings should be taken 'at rest' after sitting down and relaxing for several minutes, allowing 30 minutes rest after strenuous exercise.

Exercise or stress, of course, will raise BP readings, stress sometimes more so than even strenuous exercise. For this reason systolic blood pressure will normally have a range of about 30 in teenagers, for whom diastolic pressure will have a range of about 25. For people around the age of 60 the normal ranges are about 50 - 60 for systolic BP and about 30 for diastolic BP.

Note again that wrist meters read about 20 lower than the "gold standard" (Kowalski, 2006) sphygmomanometers and their diastolic readings are sometimes unrealistically low. Recently the author bought an excellent 'upper arm cuff' electronic BP meter for only $100 and it proved to be of professional standard and accuracy, and such meters I recommend.

Finally, I found that:

(a) Better, lower readings were obtained by resting my arm on a table, as is recommended for most BP meters.

(b) One should be as relaxed as possible, preferably for half an hour prior, and even mental stress that one is unaware of may raise readings.

(c) Cold weather may make readings higher (Kowalski, 2006).

Conclusion

My 40-day program undertaken over a decade ago worked wonders, as the BP results of Table 20.2 demonstrate.

The results for the eight-week program undertaken early in 2015 and shown in Table 20.3 were not as spectacular as BP was not so high to begin with but, nevertheless, the results were good, the reduction in RPR being the main improvement in Table 20.3.

During this period my cholesterol results were those shown in Table 20.4. The results are good, the high HDL level being of particular note and resulting from plenty of exercise.

Table 20.4. Author's cholesterol results (mg/dl) during 8-week program.

Item	Reading	Desirable
Total cholesterol	150	< 200
LDL cholesterol	42	< 100
HDL cholesterol	100	> 45
Total/HDL	1.5	< 4
Triglycerides	20	< 150

Along with the cholesterol tests of Table 20.4, I obtained a detailed blood analysis which gave OK results for many items such as haemoglobin, platelets, white cells, B12 and folate, detailed blood chemistry and thyroid function, but indicating very mild normocytic/normochromic anaemia, I believe because my diet had lapsed quite badly for a few weeks before the tests. According to Roizen's tables, the results of Table 20.4 indicate a reduction in 'real age' of -3.1 (Roizen, 2001).

Then an ECG proved OK, along with an echocardiogram, though not surprisingly considering my history, a stress echocardiogram showed a slightly enlarged heart, i.e. somewhat weakened heart muscle (cardiomyopathy), reminding me that I had been doing very little of my gym drill for a few years and consuming too much alcohol at times.

The couple of slightly negative results in these tests convinced me that I should once again undertake the 2-year program described in the next chapter.

Finally, a note of caution. One should build up one's exercise routine carefully and gradually. In the case of the infirmed, convalescent or partially disabled it might be wise, if not necessary, to avoid the risk of dropping free weights on themselves and use exercise machines which avoid such injury risks.

Chapter 21

2-Year Program to Reverse Atherosclerosis

> *For example, a male patient of mine suffered a heart attack.*
> *I recommended that he strive to halve his LDL cholesterol, take a little aspirin, a bit of wine, some vitamins, and adopt a prudent diet combined with an exercise and stress-reduction program.*
> Dr Hosen Kiat (formerly Research Director, Cedars-Sinai Medical Centre), *Eastwest Medical Makeover* (2002).

Introduction

The diet and exercise program of Chapters 17 - 19 is designed for general health and prevention of heart disease, not curing it. The program of Chapter 20, on the other hand, is designed simply to get one a little fitter as quickly as possible and it is far too short to be of any benefit in a context such as that of regression of atherosclerosis.

It takes up to 2 years of zealous diet to reduce atheroma a modest amount, if at all, and in such a special effort you should:

(1) Analyse your vascular symptoms and their causes over the years to try and establish some 'what not to do' rules.

(2) Tune your diet to:
(a) Reduce fat intake to around 10% of calories, a level that also minimizes cancer risk (Kurzweil, 1993).
(b) Keep protein intake somewhere near 20% of calories, an optimal level for most purposes (Corder, 2007).
[For athletes 30% might be more appropriate (Sears, 1995)].
(c) Consume only 'good' carbohydrate such as wholemeal bread and vegetables, limit sugar and thence fruit intake, and avoid 'bad' carbohydrate, in particular added sugar.

(3) Add the best of the natural supplements discussed in Chapters 12 - 14, namely lecithin and linseeds, omega-3 oils, niacin, L-arginine, lysine, selenium, and vitamins C , tocotrienol form E, and B complex.

(4) Try to do an hour or two of various kinds of exercise a day.

(5) Keep up this special effort for 2 years.

Upping the exercise

The aim was to do the equivalent of about 3 or more hours of walking daily to use up 800 calories daily, this exercise calories total being calculated as shown in Chapter 19. Typically, this involved:

(1) Before lunch a short calisthenics (2 minutes) and running on the spot routine (4 minutes), the latter 'knees up' about half the time.

(2) Half an hour or more road bike in the afternoon.

(3) Half an hour or more of walking during the day (for shopping or just for exercise).

(4) A continuous 30-minute circuit training drill with light weights (and thus 30 - 50 reps) and exercise bike (between each weights exercise), the weights exercises being those shown in Table 20.1.

(5) Two 5-minute periods of floor exercises each evening.

There were also usual domestic chores such as getting meals and washing clothes. Whenever half an hour or an hour was spent on a domestic task such as mowing the lawn or vacuuming the house, however, this was counted as part of the daily exercise quota.

Results for the 2-year program

The normal routine: The diet and exercise routines of preceding chapters are sound but do not add calories for exercise and tended to leave me lacking in energy. If anything, this has always helped me keep up desk work for long hours. The result was too much time in bed or a chair, ultimately a major factor in TIAs and heart symptoms.

If you can get deep vein thrombosis (DVT) sitting on a plane for 12+ hours then you can get similar problems being in bed or sedentary 90% of the time during stressful day and night book efforts. One solution is to make sure of doing some exercises around the middle of each evening.

The 2-year program (2008-2009):

Table. 21.1. Rested/relaxed BP results during various periods. Exercise levels are daily average. W = walking (240 cals/hr) R = road bike (360 cals/hr), C = calisthenics (480 cals/hr) J = jogging, CT = continuous circuit training (both 600 cals/hr).

Period	Weeks	Exercise (hours)					Exercise calories	Stress & diet	BP	
		W	R	J	C	CT			Syst	Dia.
2008A	12	0.5	1.5	0	0.1	0.15	798	OK	136.6	94.1
2008B	9	1	0.5	0	0.1	0.15	558	?	149.1	93.3
2008C	2	0.5	0.5	0	0.25	0.6	780	OK	154.0	87.7
2008D	12	0.5	0.5	0	0.25	0.6	780	OK	135.0	85.7
2008E	5	0.5	0.5	0	0.25	0.6	780	OK	118.9	76.3
2008F	6	0.5	0.5	0	0.25	0.6	780	?	134.9	75.7
2008G	6	0.5	0.5	0	0.25	0.6	780	OK	123.4	79.5
2009A	6	0.5	0.5	0	0.25	0.6	780	OK	120.6	74.1
2009B	3	0.5	0.5	0	0.25	0.6	780	?	130.9	72.4
2009C	10	0.5	0.5	0	0.25	0.6	780	OK	116.2	70.6
2009D	14	0.5	0	0.5	0.25	0.6	900	OK	110.0	66.0
2009E	19	0.5	0.25	0.25	0.25	0.6	840	OK	108.0	65.7
2010A	22	0.5	0.25	0.25	0.25	0.6	840	OK	104.6	62.8
2010B	30	1	0	0	0.25	0.65	750	OK	114.3	64.7

As shown in Table 20.2, BP had already been reduced by earlier efforts, but was reduced in Table 21.1 to unexpectedly low levels.

Note that a wrist meter was used and these read lower than sphygmomanometers. The readings in Table 21.1, and also Tables 20.2 and 20.3, have been adjusted according to comparisons of the wrist meter readings and sphygmomanometer readings taken by a specialist.

The effect of level of exercise upon BP was demonstrated in period 2008A in Table 21.1 when 1.5 hours/day road biking was done. With reduction in exercise in 2008B and some special work efforts there was a significant increase in BP, in part owing to increased alcohol consumption.

To ensure reduced BP again, therefore, an intense and continuous 30+ minute circuit training drill was done daily. Thus, after a two week initial 'recovery period' (period 2008C in Table 21.1), BP returned to a low level in period 2008D and then dropped below 120 in period 2008E. There was a slight increase in period 2008F with occasional stress and dietary lapses with return to BP circa 120 again at the end of the year (period 2008G).

With continuation of the new improved program BP results in 2009 were much better than expected, except for a period of lapse (2009B) involving an especially intense writing project. When a 30-minute jog was substituted for road biking in period 2009D, in fact, remarkably low BP resulted. Thanks to almost 2 years of increased exercise efforts, BP decreased still further in period 2009E, but only slightly, when jogging and road biking were both done, but on average every second day.

More than once Table 21.1 proves the obvious, that higher levels of exercise improve both general and vascular fitness and thence BP. As a result, therefore, with sustained higher levels of exercise systolic BP was eventually reduced to near 100 with continuation of the 2-year program for a further year (2010).

Cooke and Zimmer (2002) hold that if your blood pressure is as low as 90/60 and you can still stand up OK, this is healthy and better for your heart and blood vessels in the long run.

As I had been found by his childhood GP to have "low blood pressure" I concluded that these lower levels of BP did indicate a return of vascular function to more normal levels.

Other results

Best of all, I found a stasis ulcer episode that I had had for almost a year disappeared within only a few weeks, far quicker than the year or more that it took on two previous occasions. Indeed, such a speedy rate of recovery might be compared to the very strict Moerman cancer diet curing varicose ulcers in only 6 weeks (Jochems, 1990).

The heart pains I had had for several years took longer. Blood cholesterol can be lowered in weeks but it takes up to 6 months for blood vessel function to improve significantly (Heber, 1998) and a year or two before regressions in plaque significant enough to eliminate heart symptoms are likely to occur.

By the end of the two-year program heart symptoms, the result of clogging in the circumflex branch of the left coronary artery, were much reduced and eventually they were all but gone. In addition, the annoying neck pains (from a partially obstructed left external carotid artery*) during road bike rides had almost disappeared by the end of the first year, another sign of significant arterial improvement.

*[In late 2011 a carotid ultrasound showed calcified deposits in the left carotid artery but insignificant stenosis, suggesting that the personal efforts described in this book had almost eliminated any occlusion.]

These crucial latter two improvements were the result of long term exercise in considerable amounts, along with careful diet, perhaps the key supplement for which, in the end, was the Mohr Formula (i.e., lecithin, linseeds, lysine + vitamin C - see Chapter 2), the reasons including:

(a) Arteries became less 'sticky,' improving blood flow.
(b) Facilitation of passage of cholesterol etc. through membranes.
(c) Lecithin's role in HDL and thence reverse cholesterol transport.
(d) Reduction in LDL and increase in HDL quality and quantity.
(e) Chelation of plaques and arterial repair.

In early 2015 my diet and stress levels lapsed for several months, resulting in reappearance of stasis dermatitis on one ankle, and pains in a sizeable atheroma in my left circumflex coronary artery. I then undertook the 8-week program of Table 20.3 and this began to fix these problems, and after only about 10 weeks they had disappeared and I resolved to avoid further 'lifestyle lapses.'

Indeed, a few weeks before the latter 'fix up', I had gone through many tests as a precursor to having an angiogram. After a stress echocardiogram the specialist insisted I take 3 heart pills before he would recommend the angiogram. I refused, he argued for half an hour, but I stuck to my guns and he booked the angiogram. Then, after all the preliminary tests had been needlessly redone, I was told that I would not be allowed to go home alone after the angiogram, or live alone that first night. Used to living alone, and tired of needless bureaucratic hassle so typical of hospitals, I cancelled the angiogram – maybe another day/year?

A few weeks after the aforementioned 'fix up', the largish atheroma I had been able to feel in my LCACB (left coronary artery, circumflex branch, or 'circumflex' for brevity) ruptured, leaving a few centimeters of the artery on one or both sides of the site somewhat sore for a few days. I stuck it out without panic etc., however, and am AOK again now, and my confidence in some of the recommendations of this book remains good.

Conclusions

To combat and even reverse heart disease:

1. Eliminate excess body weight as excess weight is the most important lifestyle factor affecting heart health (Superko, 2004).

2. Limit fat calories to 10% and minimize saturated and trans fat in your diet. This limit was used in the Lifestyle Heart Trial which obtained 2% regression of relative coronary artery stenosis after one year. After 5 years 3.1% regression was obtained whereas there was 11.8% progression in the control group (Gielen et al., 2001).

The result after a year compares well with 0.8% median reduction in percent atheroma volume[1] (PAV) in coronary arteries obtained with high statin dosage in the 2-year ASTEROID trial (Nissen et al., 2006).

Other median results were -9% in atheroma volume in the worst 10 mm segment of artery and -7% in "normalized total atheroma volume."

Mean LDL levels were reduced by 53% to 61 mg/dl, and mean HDL increased by 15% to 49 mg/dl (c.f. Kurzweil's results in Table 16.2).

The Kurzweil-Ornish ultra-low 10% fat intake is also recommended by the Pritikin Longevity Centre where 83% of patients on BP medication have been able to discontinue it, 62% have been able to discontinue heart medications, and 80% have been able to avoid bypass surgery for at least five years (Gottlieb et al, 1990).

3. Include circa 20% protein to keep carbohydrates at or below 70% as higher carbohydrate levels increase triglyceride levels (Superko, 2004).

4. Limit or eliminate meat consumption and eat fish instead as mortality from ischemic heart disease is 20% lower in occasional meat eaters, 26% lower in vegans and 34% lower in people who eat fish but not meat (Key at al., 1999).

5. Limit simple sugars and alcohol to help maintain HDL2b, the type of HDL responsible for reverse cholesterol transport (Superko, 2004).

6. Include plenty of antioxidants to combat aging and disease.

---

[1] PAV = 100(A$_{int}$ - L)/A$_{int}$ with A$_{int}$ = internal cross sectional area (CSA) of artery and L = CSA of lumen (this is calculated "for the entire vessel").

Note: One large study found that changes in the whole coronary vascular tree best predict coronary events (Sdringola et al., 2006).

7. Work to get your LDL level < 100 and increase your HDL levels, *as this is when regression of cholesterol damage occurs* (McGowan, 1998). Indeed, it has been suggested that the goal should be LDL < 70 for high risk coronary patients (Nissen et al., 2006).[2] As shown in Table 16.2 the quickest way to achieve this is exercise on top of an ultra-low-fat diet.

8. Note also that TG < 150 is desirable as higher levels tend to produce especially dangerous *small dense LDL* (McGowan, 1998).

9. Take niacin in moderate to high doses to quickly reduce TG and LDL-C levels and increase HDL-C levels.

10. Take fish oil capsules with EPA and DHA to help reduce TG levels, increase HDL levels, and improve endothelial health.

11. Also take garlic to help reduce cholesterol levels.

12. Take L-arginine powder to restore NO levels and improve endothelial health (see Chapter 13).

13. Take folic acid + B_6 and B_{12} to normalize homocysteine levels.

14. Take B_1 to improve heart function.

15. Take vitamins C, E and selenium to help preserve NO. There is some evidence that vitamin E can prevent and even reverse artery clogging and also that vitamin C improves artery dilation.

16. Take 300 mg magnesium daily, especially if you have variant angina, in which case somewhat more might be helpful, if tolerable.

17. Lecithin, in line with the aims of current research, may increase HDL in both quality and quantity and thus help unclog arteries.

18. Alcohol in moderation improves artery dilation and, indeed, as noted in Chapter 6, the author has found it a life-saver in this regard.
Limit alcohol to avoid increasing triglyceride levels. Dark grape and pomegranate juices are healthy substitutes.
Aspirin and alcohol thin the blood which also helps in plaque reduction. In moderation alcohol also increases HDL, but mostly not the HDL2b responsible for reverse cholesterol transport (Superko, 2004).

---

[2] LDL circa 60 to eliminate CVD risk (30 if clinical history) has been suggested.

19. A Californian study found that regular tea drinkers had one third less coronary artery damage and two-thirds less cerebral artery damage. Tea thins the blood and reduces artery clogging by blocking thromboxane production, the tannin catechin in green tea having been found as effective as aspirin in preventing platelet aggregation (Carper, 2000).

20. Many of us are couch potatoes. To improve circulation and reduce thrombus formation do some sort of indoor exercise in the middle of every evening as well as outdoor exercises during the day.

21. Both exercise and stress reduction have been found as effective as medication in reducing heart attack risk. Stress reduction is important because mental stress releases 'fight or flight' hormones such as adrenaline which increase heart rate, blood pressure and blood lipid or 'fuel' levels. The latter are not used to any great extent and remain in the bloodstream and may contribute to arterial deposits.

Patients with heart disease, of course, often experience pain when subjected to unhealthy 'stationary stress' because it contracts coronary arteries. Some practice at relaxation techniques that can be used to cope with and recover from stressful events is therefore well worthwhile.

22. Establish a sound *maintenance* exercise routine. Effective exercise should make you at least slightly out of breath and to strengthen your heart it should get you into your target heart range (see Table 7.1).

As noted in Chapter 7, the results of the Heidelberg Regression study showed that 2000 - 2200 or more 'exercise calories' per week may give regression of heart disease, no doubt in large part because, as the results of Table 16.2 show, this level of exercise + low fat diet reduces cholesterol levels substantially.

We all know that a couple of weeks of fairly intensive exercise training or rehab work will do wonders for the body, including the vascular system. A two-year program of fastidious diet, supplements, and exercise, therefore, should do wonders!

Finally, note that:

(a) Depending upon individual circumstances the 'exercise-dosage' regimes of the foregoing program should be varied.

(b) Your heart improvement efforts should be done in consultation with a physician.

Chapter 22

CONCLUSIONS

> *Magnesium is one of the most important and healing minerals in the body. It can help prevent - - heart disease, asthma, and diabetes. It can also treat - - chronic conditions such as fatigue, mitral valve prolapse, and muscle aches and spasms.*
> Richard Firshein, *The Neutraceutical Revolution* (1998).

Brief summary

To reduce aging, and decrease heart, stroke and cancer risk:

[1] Diet:

(a) Fruits, vegetables, fish and fibre wherever possible and minimize fat, sugar, salt, caffeine and alcohol.

(b) Include foods that reduce cholesterol such as those rich in omega-3 fatty acids, phytosterols and L-arginine.

(c) Include food rich in carotenoids such as beta-carotene and lycopene, both of which are good antioxidants.

(d) Include food rich in antioxidant flavonoids such as grapes, apples, cranberries, onions, broccoli, celery and tea.

(e) Have plenty of fluids to keep your blood reasonably thin.

[2] Diet supplementation:

(a) Cholesterol reduction: Lecithin and omega-3 fish oil & garlic oil capsules.
Niacin, policosanol, or prescribed drugs on a temporary basis.

(b) Fat metabolism to assist cholesterol reduction: nicotinamide (B3).

(c) For homocysteine folate, B6, B12.

(d) Antioxidants: selenium, vitamins A, C and E.

(e) Blood thinners: aspirin, a daily drink or two of red wine.

(f) BP, heart rhythm, variant angina: magnesium.

(g) General: multivitamin & mineral tablets.

(h) For skeletal health calcium.

A simplified long-term supplements program is given in Chapter 18.

[3] **Exercise:** to reduce weight, reduce triglycerides, increase HDL, strengthen the heart, replace fat with muscle, and elasticize blood vessels.

General recommendations for the long term

[1] Diet

Long-term diet should, but for the occasional exception, stay true to the objectives of adequate fibre, minimum fat [not much above 10% of total calories and avoiding saturated fat as much as possible], minimum refined sugar and not too much alcohol, caffeine, carbohydrate or salt.

On diet, the author strongly recommends purchase of a comprehensive calorie counter book, and a book with tables giving the vitamin and mineral content of various foods.

The NHMRC now recommends just two standard drinks for both men and women and several studies have shown that this level of consumption does indeed reduce risk of heart attack and stroke for people over 45.

A group of scientists proposed a 'polymeal' that could cut heart disease risk[1] (*British Medical Journal,* 329, 2004, 1447-1450) to the point at which men could expect to live almost 7 years longer and women almost 5 years longer.

They suggested that:

(a) One 150 ml glass of red wine a day could cut risk by 32%.
(b) Eating fish four times a week cuts risks by 14%.
(c) Garlic reduces risk by 40% by lowering cholesterol levels.
(d) Eating 400 gm of fruit and vegetables a day has a smaller effect.
(e) 100 gm of dark chocolate daily can reduce blood pressure by 20%, in turn reducing heart disease risk.
(f) A handful of almonds should be included in the 'polymeal.'
(g) Eating all these foods cuts risk by a massive 75% and without the wine the risk reduction is only slightly reduced to 65%.

Like Corder (2007) I strongly disagree with (e) as this much chocolate has about 30 gm of fat, adding more than an additional 10% fat calories to the diet of Table 17.1 and increasing both heart disease and cancer risk, as the equations developed by Kurzweil and given in Chapter 16 illustrate.

---

[1] A "polypill" combining aspirin, a diuretic, and a statin, has been claimed to halve risk of stroke (diuretics lower BP & the thiazide type are vasodilators).

22. Conclusions

In the long term such an amount of fat in the diet will also increase blood cholesterol levels, in turn increasing vascular disease and clogging and thence blood pressure.

Cocoa contains antioxidant flavenols such as catechin and epicatechin which protect NO, reduce LDL oxidation, reduce platelet clumping, improve blood flow, reduce blood pressure, and may help prevent plaque buildup. A UC Davis study found that 6 weeks of cocoa consumption increased brachial artery flow by up to 76% (Nicholas J, Natural methods for reversing atherosclerosis, rejuvality.com, 2009).

Thus dark chocolate in small amounts is OK, however, and a study of 4849 people aged 35 and over, and of whom 824 ate dark chocolate regularly, found that an average of 20 grams every 3 days reduced a marker for inflammation by 17% compared with those who did not have chocolate and those who consumed larger amounts (di Guiseppe et al., *J Nutr* 138 (2008) 1939-1945).

Some authors are loath to recommend even a single standard alcoholic drink, especially to nondrinkers (McGowan, 1998). This reluctance is largely because of the increasing sociological and health problems caused by excessive consumption of alcohol.

The Australian Alcohol Guidelines recommended by medical authorities in 2006 were shown in Table 10.1. In these daily consumption levels of 2 standard drinks (SD) for women and 4 for men are suggested as "safe" in the long term.

If one is concerned about thinning the blood a little to reduce heart attack and stroke risk, therefore, a safe or 'medicinal' dosage level should be adhered to on a daily basis. Then for best cardiovascular health results this should be had in the evening in a slow and relaxed 'armchair' fashion in order to also obtain the very considerable heart health benefits of stress reduction.

Note, however, that

(a) Dark grape juice and cocoa are also good sources of antioxidants, whilst, as discussed later in this chapter, pomegranate juice is far more beneficial than red wine.

(b) The blood thinning property ascribed to alcohol can be obtained from small amounts of aspirin.

(c) A study of the data from almost 200,000 people found that those who had more than two cups of tea a day had 21% lower risk of stroke than those who drank less than one cup a day (Arab et al., *Stroke* 40 (2009) 1786-1792).

22. CONCLUSIONS

[2] Diet supplementation

Suggestions for medium term (that is, for 12 months or more) dietary supplementation are given in the final column of Table 18.1. Suggestions for dealing with heart disease were also given in Chapters 2 and 3.

Older people should take at least half an aspirin daily to dilate arteries, thin the blood, and reduce inflammation. Vitamin E also has these last two effects and aspirin + vitamin E gives better results.

Indeed, for men over 40, and post-menopausal women, half or one aspirin a day is mandatory. Aspirin is a cheap, natural and mild product from the bark of willow trees so, except in circumstances of rare intolerance, recommend half an aspirin should be taken straight after breakfast.

If you have had a heart attack and/or heart surgery it might be worth taking a magnesium tablet daily too as magnesium helps prevent arrhythmia, angina, heart attack and fatal fibrillation.

Magnesium supplements also help regress the damage that high BP can cause to the blood vessels of the retina and which may eventually affect vision (Lieberman & Bruning, 1977).

Selenium has been found to increase life expectancy and is one of a group of antioxidants which limit LDL oxidation and thus reduce heart disease (Lappenna et al., 1998). It is more effective when taken in conjunction with vitamin E which in turn is more effective taken in conjunction with vitamin C.

Thus 'SEC' is the trio of key antioxidant supplements recommended for the long term and a convenient source is 'Selenium ACE' powder which contains selenium and vitamins A, C and E, very much in line with the later versions of the Moerman cancer therapy (Jochems, 1990).

A daily garlic capsule is also recommended because garlic can reduce heart disease risk considerably. Alternatively, garlic can be introduced into the cooking of pasta, fish and vegetables.

In addition, take a comprehensive multivitamin and mineral tablet occasionally, or daily if other supplements are not had.

For those with cholesterol concerns, lecithin, niacin or Policosanol can be tried to help 'kick start' efforts at lowering blood cholesterol.

Note too that fish oil has been found to be helpful in dealing with ADHD, sometimes along with reduced dosages of Ritalin, and that lecithin might also be helpful in this regard.

Indeed, wide-ranging benefits are ascribed to lecithin (see Chapter 2), no doubt because of its ability to facilitate passage of cholesterol through cell membranes and its role in HDL and thence reverse cholesterol transport, functions which may help deal with atherosclerosis, Alzheimer's and other neurological diseases, arthritis, glaucoma and many other conditions involving infiltration of excesses of substances such as cholesterol.

The linseeds had with lecithin (see Chapter 2) are a good source of vitamin B17, a good prevention against cancer (Mohr 2012b, 2013).

[3] Exercise

Many older people, however, only do walking as a deliberate exercise and then not much of it. Upright walking places little load on most muscles and bones and a variety of other exercises such as cycling and resistance training is needed to maintain adequate strength in all parts of the whole body.

Obviously calisthenics exercises such as those of the well-known 5BX program (Penguin Books, 1964) should be done for flexibility and these should present no difficulty to all but those who are bedridden.

For strength some effort should be made at resistance exercises with modest weights and a substantial number of repetitions to give a balance of strength and endurance. Taking care to avoid doing more harm than good one should start with small weights and gradually increase the numbers of reps and the weights.

An exercise bike, of course, is very useful indeed and should be used daily for several minutes working at different intensities.

There are few better aerobic exercises than jogging but care must be taken to slowly build up distance. This can be done by jogging only from 20 to 100 metres in a single stretch at the outset, stopping for a rest, and then doing another stretch, continuing until a few stretches have been done. Ultimately the stretches can be gradually combined into a single jogging session of 10 - 20 minutes which can then be gradually extended to 30 minutes or more.

With a weight routine one should feel slight strain around halfway through a routine set of reps. At the onset of moderate strain those of us exercising for heart health should stop.

With running some measure of fatigue will appear halfway through, if not earlier, but we settle into a rhythm and should finish our routine distance fairly comfortably but a little tired afterwards.

Likewise, with walking any worthwhile distance, halfway through we might feel a little fatigue, and towards the end of a long walk we should be feeling that we are indeed beginning to test our endurance slightly.

It is, of course, very important to avoid the risk of injury or even stroke trying to push excessive weights or walk or run so far as to subject oneself to excessive strain.

A good example of the *synergistic* effects of exercise and dietary supplementation, UCLA scientists found that exercise reduced atherogenesis, and this effect was considerably increased if antioxidant vitamins C and E were also had, along with L-arginine (BBC online report 28/5/04). Clearly, exercise opens up the blood vessels and supplementary L-arginine increases protective nitric oxide (NO) levels to help keep them open, whilst antioxidants increase NO half-life.

Recommendations on heart & vascular health

[1] Blood pressure

Too many people with elevated blood pressure are given medication without any attempt to deal with the underlying cause, very often atherosclerosis. The result is usually that their arteries simply deteriorate further and a few years down the track they end up on the operating table for a bypass operation and perhaps valve replacement as well, just as the author's eldest brother did.

Note also the recent finding that the beta-blocker drug atenolol, for which 2.8 million prescriptions were issued in Australia over a recent 12 month period, was found to be no more effective than a placebo by Swedish researchers and involved a risk of death 13 times higher than did other BP-lowering medications.

Another study published in *The Lancet* found that atenolol was associated with a 26% higher risk of stroke compared to other drugs and that beta-blockers only reduced stroke risk by 19%, a smaller reduction than expected (Creswell, 2005).

As seen in Chapters 20 and 21, however, blood pressure can be reduced by careful diet and exercise within a few weeks.

Desirable BP targets are 115 for the systolic and 75 for the diastolic. Note too that systolic BP is indicative of the elasticity of one's blood vessels whereas diastolic BP is indicative of the degree of cholesterol clogging of one's circulation system.

22. CONCLUSIONS

Note here that for the ages of 60+ 1960s medical tables suggested BP "normal" ranges of 115-170/70-100 (Entwistle, circa 1965). If one is trying to *avoid* the effects of aging such as heart disease then, as Kowalski (2006) suggests, one aims for the bottom of this range.

2] Cholesterol levels

Table 22.1 shows cholesterol levels associated with various degrees of risk of cardiovascular disease. These reflect the fact that, to accommodate more adipose tissue, women have HDL levels 15 to 20% higher than men before menopause, thus being able to tolerate higher cholesterol levels safely. The author recommends a total cholesterol (TC) level of less than 180 mg/dl as most people with heart disease have a level below 240, but if you have heart disease TC $\leq$ 150 is recommended (Christensen, 2001).

Table 22.1. Cholesterol levels (mg/dl) and levels of cardiac risk.

Cardiac Risk	Men			Women		
	HDL	TC	TC/HDL	HDL	TC	TC/HDL
Very low	65	150	2.3	75	180	2.4
Low	50	200	4	65	227.5	3.5
Average	45	225	5	55	247.5	4.5
Moderate	25	250	10	40	280	7
High	<25	>300	>12	<40	>360	>9

Along with TC = 180 the author recommends a minimum HDL of 45, giving a TC/HDL ratio = 4. Indeed, HDL levels of 60 are desirable and give great cardiovascular protection. Then TC = 180 gives TC/HDL = 3, giving a comfortable safety margin within which your levels can vary a little.

A test for apolipoprotein B (apo B) can be done to indicate levels of small LDL. High levels of this are called *LDL pattern B* or ALP (atherogenic lipoprotein profile) and result in three times higher risk of heart disease. 50% of men and 30% of premenopausal women with heart disease have ALP which is often hereditary (Superko, 2004).

A test for apolipoprotein A1 (apo A1), the main protein in HDL, can be done also, the ratio apo B/apo A1 being as useful as TC/HDL for diagnosis and prognosis (Sniderman et al., 2003; Benderly et al., 2009).

Normal triglyceride levels are 10 - 190 and with high levels of exercise triglyceride levels will sometimes be almost zero.

219

As noted in Chapter 2, however, it is Lp(a) that is mainly responsible for atherosclerotic plaques and levels above 20 mg/dl are dangerous and Superko (2004) recommends 15 mg/dl as a safe level.

Niacin is a natural product that helps reduce cholesterol levels (Kowalski, 1987), including Lp(a), also increasing HDL.

Another is Policosanol which has been shown to be effective in numerous Cuban trials but a 2001 German study by Berthold et al. concluded: "Our results suggest that Policosanol is devoid of clinically relevant lipoprotein-lowering properties in white patients."

As noted in Chapter 2, lecithin has been found beneficial for a wide range of medical conditions and has been shown to lower cholesterol levels (Jiminez et al., 1990).

In 2008 British heart experts called for a family screening program to detect familial hypercholesterolemia (FH), a genetic disorder which prevents the liver from clearing cholesterol from the blood, resulting in heart attacks and strokes up to 40 years earlier than normal. Most people with FH have a single gene defect and a 50% chance of passing it to their children. Those who inherit a double defect are often dead by early adulthood. The purpose of screening was to identify children with FH so that they could be encouraged to make lifestyle choices to reduce cholesterol levels and take medication when young adults (Creswell, 2008).

[3] Reversing atherosclerosis

Along with careful diet and exercise, antioxidants such as vitamins C and E help reduce cholesterol levels (Fischer, 1989).

Note that, whilst normalizing blood cholesterol levels is important to prevent further progress of cardiovascular disease, it is also crucial to reduce cholesterol plaques as far as possible and any measure that reduces cholesterol levels significantly may give plaque regression.

McGowan (1998) suggests that regression of cholesterol damage occurs when LDL level < 100 mg/dL and that then 6 to12 months will be required for significant diminution of atherosclerotic plaques.

To achieve LDL = 100 the total cholesterol level of 180 suggested earlier requires, assuming VLDL approximately = TG/5,

HDL = 180 - 100 - TG/5 = 50   if TG (triglycerides) = 150

a 'good' HDL level for men as results of four recent trials suggested that HDL > 45 gives regression of atheroma (Nicholls et al., 2007).

22. Conclusions

Recent research has shown that HDL level is an independent predictor of CV risk and the ASTEROID trial concluded that: *"Treatment to LDL-C levels below currently accepted guidelines, when accompanied by significant HDL-C increases, can regress atherosclerosis in coronary disease patients"* (Nissen et al., 2006).

In this trial mean LDL was reduced to 61, leading to recommendations that LDL < 70 is required for optimal results, a level which, as seen in Table 16.2, can be obtained with low fat diet and exercise.

The mean result of four large statins trials (including ASTEROID) was

- 23.5% in LDL to 87.5, + 7.5% in HDL to 45.1, with regression occurring when LDL < 87.5 and HDL > 45 (Nicholls et al., 2007).

Such results make sense bearing in mind that it is estimated that primitive hunter-gatherer people had LDL of 50 - 75 mg/dL, reminding us that it is also estimated that they had about 600 mg vitamin C daily, in part the basis of the Pauling-Rath 'vitamin C theory' of heart disease.

With improved cholesterol levels, however, *"you may see a quick improvement in your health - - the endothelium can rapidly repair itself given the right ingredients. As endothelial health improves, the body is able to make more and more NO, thus improving the health of the blood vessels"* (Cooke and Zimmer, 2002).

At present, however, the best course appears to be the 10% fat calories diet, a sound regime of supplements, and a comprehensive exercise routine, as proposed in the programs of this book. Such an approach will rapidly lower BP, RPR and cholesterol levels and, given time, give you the best chance of reversing atherosclerosis.

It takes a year, however, to obtain at best regression of only about 1%, or 2%, but as noted at the close of Chapter 21, better results have been obtained using the '10% fat limit + lifestyle' approach than by using the latest statin drugs.

An example of the lesser benefits of moderate fat intake (i.e. circa 20% fat calories), a 4-year Stanford study of 300 patients with coronary artery disease found that those with low-fat diet, lipid-lowering (by medication), and exercise programs, had a decrease in minimum luminal diameter[2] of 0.024±0.067 mm/year compared with a decrease of 0.045±0.073 mm/year in the control group (Gielen et al., 2001).

---

[2] The lumen diameter of the right coronary artery is ≥ 2.5 mm.

22. Conclusions

As noted in Chapter 2, injection of phospholipids has been found to clear atherosclerotic deposits (Friedman, Byers, Rosenman, 1957).

More recently studies with a newly discovered apo A protein, apoA1 Milano, found in the HDL of genetically related people with low HDL but no history of heart disease, showed that with just five weekly infusions of this protein, together with phopholipids, percent atheroma volume (PAV) decreased by up to 1 percent (Nissen et al., 2003), so that *"artery buildups had regressed about 4 percent"* (Haney, 2005).

This is comparable to results normally obtained in 1 or 2 year trials but unfortunately the placebo was saline, not phospholipid, so how much the phospholipids contributed to the results is not known (Hegele, 2004).

The important phospholipid lecithin, which as shown in Table 2.1 is a major component of HDL, may also be of benefit in regressing atherosclerosis, perhaps in conjunction with omega-3 oils, lysine and vitamin C, as noted at the close of Chapter 2.

Pomegranate is the only food containing highly antioxidant *punicalagins* which are up to 95% absorbed and are mainly responsible for its antioxidant and health benefits, one study finding free radical activity decreased by 71% (Azadzai et al., 2005). Its antiatherogenic effects include reducing LDL levels, almost doubling levels of antioxidant enzyme paraxonase-1,[3] halving oxidation in both LDL and plaques, increasing NO levels, reducing BP, and reducing blood clotting.

In a controlled one-year human study a group given statins and BP meds had a 9% increase in carotid artery intima-media thickness,[4] but a second group given pomegranate juice as well had a 35% decrease,[5] increasing carotid artery flow velocity by 44% (Aviram at al., 2004).

Another study of cardiac patients with meds, or meds + pomegranate juice, found that after 3 months stress angina increased by 38% in the meds group and decreased by 50% in the pomegranate group. Coronary artery blood flow decreased by 17% in the meds group, but increased by 18% in the pomegranate group (Sumner et al., 2005).

As for cancer, when 50 men for whom conventional prostate cancer treatment had failed were given 8 ounces of pomegranate juice daily, PSA doubling times were quadrupled (Pantuck et al., 2006).

---

[3] Carried by HDL2b so higher levels = higher HDL2b levels and more RCT.

[4] An indicator of atherosclerosis elsewhere, especially the heart.

[5] After 3, 6 and 9 months the decrease was 13, 22, 26% respectively.

[4] Strengthening the heart

It is discouraging to note that one-third of people who have balloon angioplasty to unblock a coronary artery find that the blockage tends to return within three months. When the blockage is more severe, perhaps circa 80%, a coronary bypass operation might be indicated but this, of course, is something of a 'one-way street.'

Obviously preventative measures, therefore, are preferable. As these simply involve improved diet and exercise, themselves an improvement in lifestyle, such measures are a plus at the outset.

The benefits of improved diet, in which the author includes giving up smoking and carefully limiting alcohol consumption, are often almost immediate as feelings of improved health may appear literally overnight.

To reduce BP and RPR, however, may take a few weeks, as Table 20.3 illustrates, and to reduce BP a good deal may take a year or two, as Table 21.1 demonstrates.

Reducing serum cholesterol levels takes, of course, a few months, as illustrated in Tables 16.1 and 16.2. Then 6 - 12 months or more of further careful diet and exercise are required to significantly reduce cholesterol deposits (McGowan, 1998).

Many people with cardiovascular problems have 'let themselves go' for many years, if not decades, and will need to make a considerable effort to build up an exercise program that will take off surplus fat and rebuild long lost muscle. Along the way, of course, they will be strengthening their heart.

Here, however, great care is needed. As with any muscle, the heart will give symptoms of stress such as pain or 'tightness' and these must be carefully monitored. If they are of anything like 'sharp' and last longer than a few minutes a physician should be consulted without delay.

If, on the other hand, they are quite mild and temporary then with a few weeks and months of careful diet and exercise the symptoms should regress. For symptoms of heart discomfort or 'weakness' to disappear altogether, however, may take some years, not surprising bearing in mind the large number of years it usually takes to develop cardiovascular problems, and the 2 year program described in Chapter 21 is an example of a medium-term plan to reverse heart disease.

Should all else fail, however, prescription medications are beginning to show more promise. A 2007 paper in the American Medical Association journal reported that a study conducted on 349 patients in 9 countries proved that regression of atheroma in arteries could be achieved (Nissen et al., 2006).

Atheroma in the patients was measured using tiny ultrasound devices attached to a catheter. They were then given a high dosage of rosuvastatin (40 mg) for two years after which further ultrasound inspections showed a definite reduction in atheroma. In addition, mean LDL levels fell from 130 to 61 and mean HDL levels rose from 43 to 49.

Reducing aging

Antioxidants, together with good diet and exercise, reduce cholesterol problems and the risk of cancer, and can sometimes even reverse vascular disease and cancer. It is not surprising, therefore, that it has been found that mice and rats given more exercise and fewer calories in their diet have been found to live considerably longer.

From research at the Berkeley campus of the University of California came an even more startling result. This was that a defect in the insulin growth factor gene IGF1 increased the life of worms by a factor of three.

Extrapolating the same result to humans is difficult, if not impossible, to imagine. There is no doubt, however, about the anti-aging effect of healthy diet, much of this owing to antioxidants which reduce cholesterol oxidation and deposit buildup.

To absorb vitamin B12 properly healthy stomach cells that produce plenty of intrinsic factor (IF) are needed. IF binds to B12, hiding it from bacteria so that B12-IF receptors in the small intestine can absorb it. This process becomes less efficient at 60+ and B12 levels start to drop off, the solution being B12 supplements or occasional B12 injections.

Until relatively recently atherosclerosis was regarded as simply part of the aging process and, indeed, da Vinci's recorded observation of it given in Chapter 1 is in accord with this point of view.

Today, however, we are beginning to come to some understanding of atherosclerosis and know that antioxidants such as selenium and vitamins C and E statistically reduce the incidence of heart disease.

With age our teeth and gums deteriorate. It has been found that periodontitis increases blood levels of fibrinogen, a marker for heart disease, but that treatment reduces fibrinogen levels.

Choline is used by the body to make the important neurotransmitter acetylcholine. A deficit of this nutrient play's a role in the development of neurological disorders such as Huntington's chorea, Parkinson's disease, and Alzheimer's disease (Lieberman & Bruning, 1997).

It should not be surprising to find that healthy diet and exercise keep us younger, healthier and freer from disease. What is important here, however, is having some idea of just what sort of diet and exercise program gives best results and this is the purpose of this book.

Furthermore, not only can good diet and exercise help prevent disease, there is plenty of evidence that:

(a) Ultra-low fat diet + supplements such as amgydalin, tocotrienols, and pomegranate *punicalagins* can reduce risk of, if not *cure* cancer.

(b) *Regression* of cholesterol damage can take place if LDL levels are below 100, in turn requiring total cholesterol levels of less than about 180.

Finally, however, it must be repeated that, for best results, good dietary and exercise habits are learnt young and applied throughout life.

Failing that, the many older people who suffer cardiovascular problems stand to benefit greatly from the diet and exercise ideas discussed in this book. As Cooke and Zimmer (2002) point out, vascular disease can be reversed and major surgery avoided if action is taken before blockage of arteries is too great (that is, 80% or more).

Other studies on aging

(1) Another benefit of aspirin and other NSAIDS (non-steroidal anti-inflammatory drugs) is that taken at least twice a week for two or more years they have been found to reduce incidence of Parkinson's disease by about 50% (Wahner AD et al., *Neurology* 69 (2007) 1836-1842).

(2) In a 4-week US trial people were fed salmon fillets daily, reducing cholesterol and triglyceride levels by 17% and 40% respectively.

A later trial found that those who eat fatty fish at least once a week are 60% less likely to develop heart disease (Whitaker, 2002).

(3) The omega-3 fish oils help tackle arthritis because, as noted in Chapter 12, they have anti-inflammatory effects.

A study of 8085 people over 65 found that diets rich in omega-3 fatty acids reduced incidence of Alzheimer's disease by 60% whilst with daily consumption of fruits and vegetables the reduction was 30%, but only if they were not carriers of the ApoE4 gene which increases dementia risk (Barberger-Gateau P et al., *Neurology* 69 (2007) 1921-1930).

Another study found that eating fish at least three times a week reduced the risk of brain lesions that cause dementia and stroke by 26%, while fish once a week gave a 13% lesser risk (Vitanen JK et al., *Neurology*, 71 (2008) 439-446). As noted in Chapter 15, lecithin has also been found helpful in treatment of various brain-related ailments.

(4) Some claim that antioxidants protect against CHD and cataracts, and slow aging and progress of Parkinson's disease (Lee and Lee, 1994).

Research at UC Berkeley found that the tocotrienol forms of vitamin E, especially alpha-tocotrienol, reduce the oxidation-induced brain cell death responsible for a number of age-related brain diseases (*J Biological Chemistry*, April 2000).

(5) A preliminary study of mice with a form of Parkinson's disease found that cholesterol-lowering drugs inhibited progression of the disease (Ghosh et al., *J Neuroscience* 29 (2009) 13543-13556).

A study of 1130 elderly people published in 2011 in *Archives of Neurology* found that those with higher HDL levels had lesser risk of developing Alzheimer's disease.

Trials have recently begun to test the effectiveness of testosterone + fish oils in treating Alzheimer's disease.

(6) Supplements that help dilate blood vessels may help not only heart function, but also brain function. A study published in 2010 in the journal *Nitric Oxide* found that people given a diet high in nitrate had increased blood flow in the frontal lobes of their brains, suggesting that dietary nitrate may be helpful in treating ailments such as dementia.

(7) Older people are often more prone to depression. Research combining the results of 11 studies of 15,315 people found that low blood folate levels increased the risk of depression by 55% (Gilbody S et al., *J Epidemiology and Community Health* 61 (2007) 631-637).

A recent Oxford University study found that people with Alzheimer's disease tend to have low levels of folate and vitamins B6 and B21, resulting in higher homocysteine levels. In such people brain shrinkage occurs at a much greater rate than the normal level of about 0.5% per year in old age (see Chapter 16).

(8) A 5-year study of 197 people with an average age of 75 published online in *Archives of Internal Medicine* found that the 33% who were most active had a 91% lesser risk of cognitive impairment compared to the 33% who exercised least.

(9) Noting how muscle mass decreases drastically in men after middle age, one cannot help but wonder whether minimal hormonal therapy might not be worthwhile and might not also be of benefit to the heart.

An Australian study published in 2007 in the Journal of Clinical Endocrinology and Metabolism showed that testosterone therapy for 60 men 55 and over with low testosterone levels increased testosterone levels while levels dropped in a control group. The therapy increased muscle mass and decreased abdominal fat, suggesting a promising approach to treating diabetes and heart disease in older men.

(10) A small trial found that testosterone treatment reduced brain deterioration in the most common relapsing-remitting form of multiple sclerosis by 67%, also increasing muscle mass (Sicotte NL, et al., *Arch. Neurol.* 64 (2007) 683-688). Testosterone may also be used to treat hypogonal males or for contraceptive purposes (Williams, 1998).

Both studies (9) and (10) are evidence that hormone therapy can be beneficial in reducing and even reversing aging processes.

(11) Common baldness is called androgenic alopecia and is caused by genetic sensitivity to an androgen (male sex hormone) called dihydrotestosterone (DHT) which causes the hair follicle to shrink and die.

Minoxidil, the active ingredient in Rogain, is a vasodilator which slows this process by increasing capillary circulation in the scalp and presumably other vasodilating substances such as niacin might also be helpful.

(12) Another factor in baldness may be lack of oestrogen in the scalp, and oestrogen creams might be helpful in preventing baldness.

It is interesting to note that a three-year UK clinical trial in which 200+ males were given 6 gm lysine, 6 gm vitamin C, and 800 IU vitamin E, found atherosclerotic plaque progression almost eliminated but also that several individuals began regrowing their hair (Ellis, 2005).

Reversing heart disease

Minimizing aging and heart disease requires comprehensive diet, supplementation and exercise programs, the key requirements being:

(1) Restriction of fat calories to 10%.

(2) A low GI diet rich in vegetables and fruit.

A study published in 2011 in the journal *Archives of Internal Medicine* found that among 15,318 US adults 20 years and older, those with the highest blood alpha-carotene concentrations had 39% less risk of death compared with those with the lowest concentrations. Alpha-carotene is found in many fruits and vegetables.

22. Conclusions

As far back as 1980 it was authoritatively estimated that diet might be the greatest single factor in cancer mortality and account for 35% of all cancer deaths. Doubtless it is both the overall balance of the diet and how rich it is in vitamins and other vital nutrients that are helpful, and the same applies to heart disease.

(3) Supplementation with fish oil, antioxidants [C, E (including tocotrienols) and punicalagins], lecithin, amygdalin, aspirin etc.

(4) An 'all purpose' supplement such as lecithin to reduce cholesterol and other deposits in the body and thus tackle a wide range of diseases.

For those mainly concerned with atherosclerosic heart disease, the 'Mohr Formula' of lecithin and linseeds, plus lysine and vitamin C (see Chapter 2) might be a better option.

Along with reducing LDL to circa 70 mg/dL, the focus of current research is also increasing both quantity and quality of HDL to reverse atherosclerosis. The lecithin phospholipids form part of HDL, as shown in Table 2.1, and may help achieve all these objectives.

(5) A comprehensive exercise and relaxation program. As one-time hunter-gatherers, our eyes were designed for far-field vision, not reading books, so for most of us appropriate exercises such as shifting focus from a few inches to a few feet repetitively might also be advantageous (Brookes-Simpkins, 1968).

Curing heart disease, on the other hand, may require much greater effort. Atherosclerotic plaques grow and multiply at an exponential rate (Rath, 2001b), because, as the arteries deteriorate and become more 'sticky,' Lp(a), LDL etc. become stuck to or in them at an accelerating rate.

Thus, slowing progression, and halting it if possible, takes at least 6 to 12 months, if not more, and only then might regression occur.

The Mohr Formula for heart disease is discussed in Chapters 2 and 3, whilst a detailed list of recommendations on curing heart disease is given at the end of Chapter 21.

Prevention is far easier than cure, and cure is generally a slow process, requiring two years to obtain reversal of atherosclerosis.

Conclusion

A recent study of 2300 heart disease patients published in the *New England Journal of Medicine* found no difference in the death rates of those given drugs and those given drugs and angioplasty[6] (*The Australian*, March 28, 2007). More disturbing, one 8-year follow-up study found that, except for high-risk patients with 3-vessel disease and low ejection fraction in echocardiogram tests, mortality rates were very nearly twice as high for those who'd had bypass, 32.2%, compared to those treated conservatively, 16.8% (Whitaker, 2002).

This should remind us that many heart experts such as Cooke (Cooke & Zimmer, 2002) and Kiat (2002) feel medication, whether for BP or cholesterol levels, can also be avoided in most cases.

Recently three Australian doctors said that taking statins gives the *"illusion of protection"* from heart disease and stroke and involves risk of harmful side-effects, and that many patients would be better off improving their diet, for example by eating more nuts and olive oil (Herald Sun, Melbourne, 21/1/2015).

The Mohr Plan is a *natural* diet and exercise plan aimed at achieving some regression in vascular disease and to reduce cancer risk that may have been increased by earlier bad habits like smoking or bad diet.

Indeed, Elizabeth Somers' book *The Origin Diet* (2001) argues the case for a 'natural' diet well and many of its food recommendations correspond to those in the better books on heart health and cancer prevention by diet.

Of course it has to be realized that our ancient ancestors were forced to have a natural diet, though perhaps a somewhat hit or miss one. They did not have life-saving things like antiseptics, anaesthetics and antibiotics, however, so the life expectancy of Stone Age man was only about 30.

Some of the reasons that we live longer might be evolutionary, for example a study of the data on over 3 million people and published in the *European Heart Journal* in 2010 showed that short people (less than 160.5 cm) were 1.55 times more likely to die from heart disease than tall

---

[6] After angioplasty restenosis often occurs before long. Drug-eluting stents (DES) and antiplatelet drugs are used to prevent this. Often, however, the latter have to be discontinued to allow noncardiac surgery, running a slight risk of late stent thrombosis (LAST) caused by medium sized vulnerable plaques. Despite low incidence, LAST has a high mortality rate (Karin et al., 2010).

people (more than 173.9 cm). The reason for this might be that the coronary arteries of short people are smaller in diameter and thus clog more easily.

Can diet really make a big difference? A study of mice on a calorie-restricted diet since birth showed that they lived 40% longer than mice fed normally. A 20 year follow-up study done at the University of Wisconsin on dozens of macaque monkeys showed that a healthy diet but with 30% less calories than usual cut risk of age-related diseases including diabetes and cancer by a factor of 3 and even improved brain function.

Few people can tolerate 30% calorie restriction and in laboratory animals calorie restriction is not effective when not initiated until later in life (Corder, 2007).

Alternatively, therefore, antioxidant substances such as resveratrol can be used to give similar benefits to those of calorie restriction (*The Weekend Australian,* 11-12, July 2009).

Cutting calories by, say, 10% is highly practical in the long term, however, and this should reduce your weight to about 5% below figures recommended for your height and build, perhaps a relatively optimal amount from the point of view of longevity. Then cutting fat calories to 10% also may well give very significant health and longevity prospects.

As well as a sound diet, it is also important to have regular exercise, relaxation, and sleep. Thus the present book covers all the key points in Roizen's book on staying young and healthy, *Real Age.*

You should, of course, only use the Mohr Plan as a starting point and then augment it to suit your own preferences.

Indeed, this book will have achieved its purpose even if you find just one key idea, such as realizing that you *can* do something about a history of cardiovascular, cerebrovascular or peripheral vascular symptoms because they are usually caused by cholesterol accumulation beginning in childhood, not by fate.

Alternatively, you may have some history of atherosclerotic heart disease (ASHD) in your family. If so, I hope you gain a little insight into the causes and remedies for heart disease and perhaps follow some of the advice on diet and exercise, and such key supplements as magnesium, lecithin, and selenium, to help reduce aging and your heart disease and also cancer risk.

For best results, however, you should start right away.

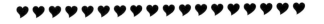

Appendix A

COMPUTER ANALYSIS OF DIET

Computer analysis of diet

For the diet of Tables 17.1 and 17.2 the results obtained using the computer program *Now You're Cooking* (Food for Thought Software, 1999) are shown in Table A.1.

Table A.1. Computer analysis of diet.

Item	Basic diet			Variation		
	mass	% mass	% cals	mass	% mass	% cals
water (g)	6811.4	94.2		7103	94.4	
calories	1694			1605		
total fat (g)	21.7	0.30	13	15.0	0.20	9
sat. fat (g)	5.3	0.07	3	3.4	0.05	2
mono fat (g)	7.8	0.11	5	5.0	0.07	3
poly fat (g)	6	0.08	4	4.5	0.06	3
cholesterol (mg)	69.4	0.001		38.6	0.001	
protein (g)	74.6	1.03	19	48.9	0.65	13
sodium (mg)	2307	0.03		2672	0.04	
carbohydrate (g)	260	3.60	68	287	3.82	78
dietary fibre (g)	26.8	0.37		35.3	0.47	
ash (g)	14.8	0.20		16.1	021	

For the %mass figures the program gave only integer results for water (95), protein (1), and carbohydrate (4), so a spreadsheet was used to give the more detailed %mass figures in Table A.1.

The calorie, fat and fibre totals are close to those of Tables 17.1 and 17.2 but the protein and carbohydrate totals are a little lower because the program uses American data, not Borushek's Australian data (Borushek, 2014).

Only 20 - 25% of fat intake is saturated fat and cholesterol intake is well under the recommended limit of 300 mg (Borushek, 2014; Cooper, 1996).

The sodium values are higher than those calculated manually in Tables 17.1 and 17.2 from data in food labeling because quantities of ingredients heavy in salt like bread and baked beans tended to be overestimates in the program's US data which is of a more 'general' nature.

Nutrient analysis

Table A.2. Analysis of dietary vitamin & mineral content.

Item	Basic diet	Variation	RDI *
calcium (mg)	641	678	800 - 1200
phosphorus (mg)	1320	1178	1000
iron (mg)	29.6	27.7	10 - 20
potassium (mg)	4842	5229	2800 - 3200
magnesium (mg)	568	566	400
zinc (mg)	8.2	10.3	12 - 15
copper (mg)	2.1	2.55	2
manganese (mg)	18.8	18.2	5 - 5.5
vitamin A (IU)	15730	12820	5000
vitamin E (IU)	6.51	5.93	15
thiamin (mg)	1.76	2.12	1.1 - 1.5
riboflavin (mg)	2.85	2.8	1.3 - 1.7
niacin (mg)	29.4	20.6	20
pantothenic acid (mg)	3.9	3.8	5 - 10
vitamin B6 (mg)	3.21	2.275	2
folate (mcg)	609	708	400 - 600
vitamin B12 (mcg)	2.66	0.96	2 - 2.4
vitamin C (mg)	54.8	173	60

* NHMRC 2009, Lieberman & Bruning (1997), Somer (2001).

Table A.2 shows the results from the *Now You're Cooking* program for the vitamin and mineral content of the example diet of Tables 17.1 and 17.2.

Recommended daily calcium intake is 800 - 1200 mg, the lower figure for men, the higher for women, and the diet is close enough to this, given that it was for the author (a man).

The diet is OK for phosphorus, iron, potassium, magnesium, copper, manganese, thiamin (B1), riboflavin (B2), niacin (B3), B6, folate and vitamins A and C.

It is borderline on zinc and pantothenic acid, and a little low on vitamin E, a shortfall easily rectified with occasional multivitamin tablets.

There is a distinct shortfall in vitamin B12 because of the lack of meat in the diet. This too can be rectified with multivitamin tablets.

Finally, note that dietary requirements for adults vary slightly with sex and age and dietary requirements for children are considerably different from those for adults, especially for children less than 7 (NHMRC, 1991).

An alternative diet

The diet shown in the following table (Table A.3) was that adopted by the author to tackle long-standing heart symptoms (Mohr, 2012b, 2013).

Some of the measures he took to minimize fat and otherwise make the diet sounder included:

[1] Noting that saturated fats tend to be those which are solid at room temperature (Christensen, 2001) the margarine had on wholemeal toast in the evening was replaced with jam, Vegemite or tomato slices. When occasionally having a couple of sandwiches for a quick lunch the same fillings were used without margarine or butter.

[2] For the tuna dish, tuna in vegetable oil had been used. Noting a report that some types of vegetable oil can lead to blindness in old age, tuna in water was used instead, stir fried with boiled rice and vegetables in a nonstick pan.

[3] Low GI raw peanuts were included with an evening tipple of two glasses of port wine. These are rich in healthy monounsaturated oils (Carper, 2000) and are also a source of L-arginine which aids the NO (nitrous oxide) production that Nobel prize winning work has shown helps prevent and even reverse atherosclerosis (Cooke & Zimmer, 2002).

[4] Wholemeal bread and fruit, either fresh, dried or as juice, replaced biscuits and cake as snacks.

Table A.3. Example diet, P = protein, C = carbohydrates, Na = sodium.

Meal	Food	Cals	P gm	C gm	Fat gm	Fibre gm	Na mg
B/fast	3 wheat biscuits + skim milk	220	12	40	1.5	12	150
	orange juice (200 ml)	80	0.5	20	0	0	10
Lunch	French onion soup + 1 slice wholemeal toast	90	6	15	1	2	200
	pasta + vegies +dilute sauce	250	9	50	1.5	1	110
	1L tea + sugar/skim milk	40	1	8	0	0	50
Dinner	Tomato soup + slice toast	155	8	25	1.5	3	500
	100 gm tuna + 125 gm rice + vegies + Worcestershire sauce	300	25	45	1.5	2	435
	125 gm peaches in light syrup	80	0.5	20	0	3	0
	0.8L tea + sugar/skim milk	30	1	8	0	0	50
Day snacks	0.5L pot of weak Ovaltine + dash sugar & skim milk	70	1	12	1	0	70
	1 medium banana or large orange + 30 gm dried fruit	160	2	40	0	6	0
	200 ml fruit juice (mixed)	90	0.5	20	0	0	0
Night snacks	0.5L pot of weak Ovaltine + dash sugar & skim milk	70	1	12	1	0	70
	2 slices wholemeal toast & jam or a tomato sandwich	220	6	45	2	4	350
	Two 30 ml glasses port wine	170	0	45	0	0	0
	30 gm unsalted peanuts	175	10	7	15	5	5
TOTAL		**2200**	**83.5**	**412**	**26**	**38**	**2000**
Percentage of total calories			**15.1**	**74.9**	**10.6**		
Dinner variation	1/2 tin low salt baked beans + 125 gm mixed veg. [main course]	250	12	45	1	15	450
TOTAL		**2150**	**70.5**	**412**	**25.5**	**51**	**2015**
Percentage of total calories			**13.1**	**76.6**	**10.7**		

For the author's height of almost 6'2" the minimum weight for a small frame is 73 kg, at his age requiring 2160 calories for a male, but another 300 calories is needed to sustain a moderate level of physical activity (Borushek, 2006). Without these additional calories, therefore, he lost weight gradually.

The primary goal of the diet was to satisfy the Kurzweil-Ornish-Pritikin 10% fat calories limit (Kurzweil, 1993) and this is very nearly achieved in Table A.3, a satisfactory result insofar as more than half the fat intake is healthy fat from peanuts.

Average protein intake is around the middle of the recommended range of 50 - 100 gm daily and also satisfies the long-standing rule that one gm of protein should be had for each kg of body weight.

Average carbohydrate intake is just above the range of 50 - 70% of total calories sometimes recommended, a situation difficult to avoid with an ultra-low fat diet.

Average fibre intake is above the 30 to 40 gm range recommended. In any case, with an ultra-low fat diet the fibre question is not quite so important as one is not counting on fibre to help reduce absorption of fat.

Sodium intake is below the 2300 mg limit suggested by the NHMRC and the USFDA. To reduce to the American Heart Association 1500 mg limit the salty soups can be omitted and sodium-reduced bread used.

Computer analysis of diet

For the diet of Table A.3 the results from the *Now You're Cooking* program were those shown in Table A.4, again using a spreadsheet to obtain more detailed %mass figures.

The calorie, protein and fibre totals are close to those of Table A.3 but the fat totals are a little higher because the program uses American data, not Borushek's Australian data (Borushek, 2014).

Only 22% of fat intake is saturated fat and cholesterol intake is well under the recommended limit of 300 mg (Borushek, 2014; Cooper, 1996).

The carbohydrate results are reasonably close to those of Table A.3, and slightly above the desirable limit of 70% because protein intake is a little less than the desirable 20% value.

The sodium values are higher than those calculated manually in Table A.3 from data in food labeling because quantities of ingredients heavy in salt like bread and baked beans tended to be overestimates in the program's US data which is of a more 'general' nature.

Table A.4. Computer analysis of diet.

Item	Basic diet			Variation		
	mass	% mass	% cals	mass	% mass	% cals
water (g)	5268	90.3		5334	90.2	
calories	2166			2155		
total fat (g)	32.2	0.6	13.4	30.5	0.5	12.7
sat. fat (g)	7	0.1	2.9	6.6	0.1	2.8
mono fat (g)	12.3	0.2	5.1	11.6	0.2	4.8
poly fat (g)	9.0	0.2	3.7	8.5	0.1	3.5
cholesterol (mg)	83.9	0.001		46.1	0.001	
protein (g)	78.7	1.3	14.5	67	1.1	12.4
sodium (mg)	2895	0.05		3329	0.06	
carbohydrate (g)	390	6.7	72.1	403	6.8	74.8
dietary fibre (g)	38.4	0.7		51.4	0.9	
ash (g)	21.1	0.4		23.2	0.4	

Nutrient analysis

Table A.5 shows the results from the *Now You're Cooking* program for the vitamin and mineral content of the example diet of Table A.3.

Recommended daily calcium intake is 800 - 1200 mg, the lower figure for men, the higher for women, and the diet is close enough to this, given that it was for the author (a man).

The diet is OK for phosphorus, iron, potassium, magnesium, copper, manganese, thiamin (B1), riboflavin (B2), niacin (B3), pantothenic acid, B6, folate and vitamins A and C.

It is borderline on zinc and a little low on vitamin E, a shortfall easily rectified with an occasional multivitamin tablet.

There is a distinct shortfall in vitamin B12 because of the lack of meat in the diet. This too can be rectified with multivitamin tablets.

Finally, note that dietary requirements for adults vary slightly with sex and age and dietary requirements for children are considerably different from those for adults, especially for children less than 7 (NHMRC, 1991).

Table A.5. Analysis of dietary vitamin & mineral content.

Item	Final diet	Variation	RDI *
calcium (mg)	673	763	800 - 1200
phosphorus (mg)	1567	1584	1000
iron (mg)	32.7	32.8	10 - 20
potassium (mg)	5002	5614	2800 - 3200
magnesium (mg)	676	718	400
zinc (mg)	12.1	14.6	12 - 15
copper (mg)	3.27	3.67	2
manganese (mg)	14.0	14.6	5 - 5.5
vitamin A (IU)	12200	15353	5000
vitamin E (IU)	8.8	8.68	15
thiamin (mg)	2.18	2.56	1.1 - 1.5
riboflavin (mg)	2.55	2.69	1.3 - 1.7
niacin (mg)	34.2	29.0	20
pantothenic acid (mg)	4.83	4.71	5 - 10
vitamin B6 (mg)	3.15	3.35	2
folate (mcg)	591	658	400 - 600
vitamin B12 (mcg)	1.84	0.79	2 - 2.4
vitamin C (mg)	192	208	60

* NHMRC 2009, Lieberman & Bruning (1997), Somer (2001).

The example diet passes most tests, in particular having calories from fat close to the minimal 10% figure suggested by Kurzweil (1993) to minimize cancer risk and normalize cholesterol levels. This is despite around half the fat coming from peanuts which are deliberately had for their health benefits.

Note, however, that it gives only enough calories for a basic level of physical activity for somebody of the author's sex, size and age. For even moderate levels of physical activity around 300 more calories are needed unless one is trying to lose weight (Borushek, 2014).

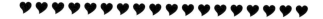

APPENDIX A: COMPUTER ANALYSIS OF DIET

Appendix B

FEM MODEL OF FLOW OBSTRUCTION

Finite element analysis of fluid flows

The *Finite Element Method* (FEM) is much used in engineering analysis (Mohr, 1992), including in biomechanics to model the stresses in various parts of the body and in prostheses for it such as artificial heart valves. A simple example of application of FEM to biomechanics is to the analysis of hydrodynamic lubrication and thence to the operation of joints in the human body (Mohr, 1982).

A good example of the application of FEM is to model the flows and pressures in a network of blood vessels. Then, to simulate the effect of obstruction in some of the vessels in the network by cholesterol plaques their 'resistance' parameters are increased.

As one might expect, the flow in the obstructed vessels decreases and that in the rest increases, resulting in larger flows and pressure in the rest or, in the present context, higher blood pressure (BP).

Here we shall use the analogy of a traffic flow network where obstructions are placed in minor streets to inhibit flow and extra lanes are added to major *arterial* roads to increase their capacity.

Then if we apply Ohm's Law of electricity we have

$$P_2 - P_1 = FR$$

where P_1 and P_2 are the potentials or *pressures* at each end of a street, F is the current or rate of flow in the street and R is the 'resistance' of the street, a function of its width, length and quality.

If we obstruct or make a street narrower, that is increase resistance R, we increase the pressure difference $(P_2 - P_1)$ between its ends. The pressure has to start at some base level so the result is an increase in the maximum pressure level 'upstream' in the network, in our current context an increase in BP.

In other words, high BP has this simple cause, that is, *obstruction* of the blood vessels by cholesterol deposits. In the case of very fine capillaries such obstruction may affect the brain and result in senile dementia of the Alzheimer type (SDAT) and ultimately in congestive stroke. In the heart atherosclerosis can weaken the heart muscle, ultimately resulting in fibrillation when the muscles work in a more nearly torsional mode and pumping ceases.

Less seriously, it may affect almost any part of the body including the eyes, for example, resulting in visibly obstructed superficial capillaries called *spiders*. More obviously, there may be obstruction of the perforating veins in the legs that connect the deep and superficial veins, resulting in *stasis dermatitis* and *stasis ulcers*.

Myself, I had two attacks of stasis ulceration on an ankle, the first of these occurring a few months before I realized the cause was indeed atherosclerosis and began developing the diet and exercise plans of this book. Both attacks proved slow to heal but would have simply got worse had I not begun improved diet and exercise routines.

An example of blockage in a flow network

Figure B.1 shows an example of the author's wide-ranging work on the Finite Element Method (Mohr, 2005). The diagram shows a simple traffic network with hourly vehicle flows into and out of the *nodes*.

All the routes connecting the nodes have a *jam density* (*JD*) or limiting capacity of 100 vehicles per km, except for routes 2-5 and 5-8 which have $JD = 300$ vehicles/km. All routes have a maximal *free flow velocity* $F_f = 60$ km/hour and length $L = 1$ km, from which the 'resistance' of each route is calculated as $R = L / F_f JD$ and used to form a 2 X 2 'element matrix.'

When the problem is solved by the finite element method (FEM) the 2 X 2 matrices for each element are deployed in a 9 X 9 system matrix (Mohr, 2014). The resulting simultaneous equations are then solved to determine the potentials at each node, from which the traffic flow velocities and densities in each element are then calculated. Setting the datum potential at node 8 as zero, the potential 'upstream' at node 2 turns out to be 0.333.

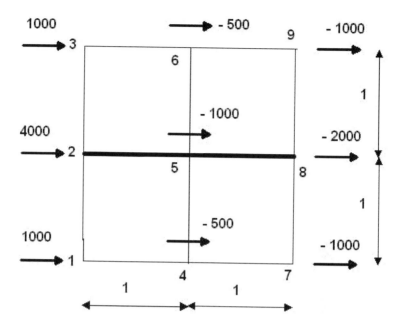

Figure B.1. Traffic flow network.
(a) JD = 100 in all routes except = 300 in 2-5 & 5-8
(b) Reduce JD in 6-9 & 4-7 to 50

If the jam densities in routes 6-9 and 4-7 (notionally arteries in the lower body in the blood flow context) are reduced to 50 the potential (pressure in our blood flow context) at node 2 (in the upper body) increases by 0.027 or about 10% to 0.360. In contrast, the potential or pressure 'downstream' at nodes 7 and 9 (in the lower body) decreases by 0.031 or about 100% from -0.030 to -0.061.

Thus our traffic flow example demonstrates the results of partial blockage in elements of a total system quite well.

If the jam density in route 5-8 is also decreased to 200 the potential at node 2 rises further to 0.417, demonstrating that when blockage extends to major arteries blood pressure rises even higher.

The situation is even worse if we realize that the quantity of flow in water pipes is proportional to the pipe diameter raised to a power of about 2.7. If we assume the same figure for blood vessels then halving the diameter of a blood vessel reduces blood flow by 85%, not just by 50% as some might guess, or by 75% as calculation based on the change in cross-sectional area would predict.

Finite element modeling of flow obstruction

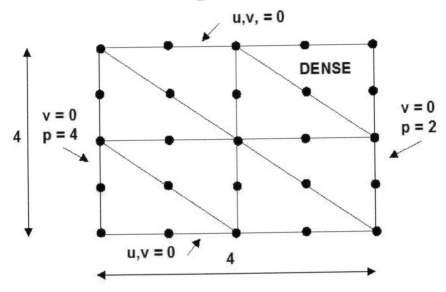

Figure B.2. Finite Element model of viscous flow.
The 'DENSE' element has 100 times the viscosity of the others.

Figure B.2 shows a Finite Element model of viscous fluid flow in a section of pipe modeled as a rectangular region (Mohr, 1992). Here the region is divided into a 'mesh' of triangular elements with six 'nodes', the whole region having 25 nodes, each with 3 *degrees of freedom* which are horizontal flow velocity u, vertical flow velocity v, and pressure p.

Nodal pressures of 4 and 2 are specified at inlet and outlet respectively to 'force' the flow. These pressure values act as 'loads' on the system and its response is determined by integrating the Navier-Stokes equations (Yuan, 1967) to calculate 18 X 18 'response matrices' for each element and adding each of these to a 75 X 75 'system matrix' and solving the resulting set of 75 simultaneous equations by Gauss reduction (Mohr, 1992).

If all elements have the same viscosity there is a linear pressure gradient in the horizontal direction and the flow is 'uniform', so that at each vertical cross section the flow has a parabolic profile such that the velocity at the top and bottom of the field is zero (as specified), 0.75 at quarter and three-quarter height, and 1.0 at mid-height.

If the viscosity of the element marked 'DENSE' at the top right of the field has 100 times the viscosity of the others, on the other hand, the flow is no longer 'uniform' and velocities near the left side are reduced by about 50%, velocities near the obstructed right side are reduced by about 90%, and the pressures within the region are increased by about 10% and no longer have a 'neat' linear gradient from inlet to outlet.

These figures are, very approximately, the sort of results that will occur when a blood vessel is obstructed, that is, flow velocities are greatly reduced and the pressures increase but less markedly. A 10% increase in blood pressure is significant, however, and 20% more so. Much more than this, of course, can be a serious problem.

Note too that Figure B.2 considers only a section of flow. When a number of blood vessels are obstructed, of course, increases in 'upstream' blood pressure are much greater, as was demonstrated using the network model of Figure B.1.

Conclusion

As demonstrated by the model of Figure B.1, 'downstream' partial blockages caused by atherosclerotic plaques increase upper body blood pressure, putting the heart and brain at risk, while reducing pressures in the extremities, resulting in peripheral vascular disease (PVD).

As might be expected, reduced blood flow rates further encourage increased deposition of lipids, resulting in new fatty streaks, or increase in the size of fibro-lipid plaques. In other words, plaque formation tends to occur at an accelerating rate at later stages (Murell et al., 2011).

Such *atherosclerosis can* affect all blood vessels, ranging from the smallest capillaries to the major arteries. Blockage of blood vessels in the brain can cause stroke, and blockage of coronary arteries can cause heart attack.

Atherosclerosis can also prevent oxygen reaching blood vessel walls so that they become anoxic and harden, a process called *arteriosclerosis*. These hardened blood vessels become weaker and may develop aneurysms. Often these aneurysms burst, in the brain causing stroke, and in major arteries in the chest region death by haemorrhage.

Elsewhere in the body, issues of 'flow' and efficiency thereof are also important. For example, food should remain in the body for only 12-18 hours before the colon eliminates it as waste. "Most British adults, however, retain waste for two to seven days – with disastrous results for their health" (Gittleman, 2005). The problem is that, the longer waste products stay in the colon, the more chance for toxins to get into the bloodstream and end up as toxic residues in body fat.

Finite elements can also be used to model the heart itself, and this can be done using flat triangular elements to approximate the curved somewhat spherical shape of the heart, or a part of it. Doubly curved elements have also been developed for this purpose, for example a 30 degree of freedom thick shell element developed by Mohr (1981, 1992).

The loading will, of course, be an internal pressure, and apertures must be included corresponding to the major arteries and veins that enter and leave the heart.

To model cardiomyopathy some of the elements are assigned lower strength parameters so that they will take up less of the 'load' on the heart but will, however, be more severely stressed compared to their reduced strength.

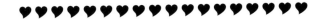

Glossary

Note: words in italics are defined elsewhere in this glossary.

ABCA1. ATP-binding membrane cassette transporter A1, a transmembrane *protein* encoded by the ABCA1 gene. ATP = *adenosine triphosphate*. Also called the *cholesterol* efflux regulatory protein (CERP). Along with ABCG1 provides a pathway for *reverse cholesterol transport*.

Acetylcholine. Neurotransmitter which plays a role in arterial contraction and in mental function.

Acetyl-L-carnitine (ACL) boosts energy production in the brain, improves the brain's glutamate receptors which are responsible for learning, and may stop formation of lipofucian, an "age spot" in neurons that interferes with memory (Gottlieb, 2000).

Adenosine triphosphate (ATP). The energy-rich ATP molecule acts as a chemical energy carrier and a coenzyme for many biological processes.

ADMA. Asymmetric dimethyl arginine. An amino acid which blocks the production of *NO* (nitric oxide) and thus has a negative effect comparable to those of cholesterol and *homocysteine*.

ALA. Alpha-linolenic acid. The form of omega-3 fatty acid found in plants which is "biologically inferior" (Wikipedia 2009) to, and hasn't the "same specific benefits" as, DHA and EPA from fish (Superko, 2004). GLA, gamma-linolenic acid, is the omega-6 plant fatty acid.

ASHD. Atherosclerotic heart disease.

Aerobic exercise. Exercises such as walking and running which use oxygen to burn sugar and body fat.

Amino acids. Organic compounds from which *proteins* are made.

Amygdalin. Nitriloside compound obtained from many plant sources, for example, apricot kernels, linseed meal, and bitter almonds. Often called vitamin B17. Has been used widely with good results to treat cancer. Sometimes confused with laetrile which is a similar but semi-synthetic compound.

Anaerobic exercise. Short bursts such as sprinting and weightlifting.

Angina pectoris. Chest pain resulting from inadequate blood flow and thence oxygen delivery to the heart, typically resulting from coronary artery blockages. Pain may also be felt in the arm, jaw or neck. See also *variant angina*.

Angiogenesis. The ability to grow blood vessels. It is a common feature of cancerous tissue. Angiogenesis in breast tissue is thought of as a sign that breast cancer may follow (Mosby's Medical Encyclopaedia, 1995).

Angioplasty. Opening up of a coronary artery using a thin catheter carrying a small balloon.

Anoxic. Deprived of adequate oxygen.

Antioxidants. Substances that can neutralize *free radicals*. In the bloodstream this helps prevent oxidation of *cholesterol*. In the cell membrane this helps prevent damage and thence protects against viral invasion. Within the cell this helps prevent mutation.

Apolipoprotein (a)/Apoprotein (a), or apo(a). Atherogenic protein unique to *lipoprotein (a)* particles (which also carry *apoB100*).

Apolipoprotein A1 or apoA1. Approx. 70% of the protein in *HDL*. Cardioprotective. Activates *lecithin-cholesterol acyltransferase* (LCAT). The apoA1 Milano mutation discovered in genetically related people in Italy is especially protective against atherosclerosis.

Apolipoprotein B or apoB. There are two types, relatively 'cardio neutral' apoB48 found in *chylomicrons*, and atherogenic apoB100 found in *LDL* and *VLDL*. ApoB48 is produced in the intestines and has 48% of the molecular weight of apoB100 which is produced in the liver.
Apo B is an integral protein, the other apoproteins being peripheral.

Apolipoprotein C. Found in *HDL*, *VLDL* and *chylomicrons*. Has types apoC1, apoC2 and apoC3 which control certain lipid transformations, apoC3 having some atherogenic effect.

Apolipoprotein D or apoD. Found in *HDL*. Forms complexes with LCAT so may be involved in transport of esterification products.

Apolipoprotein E or apo E. A *protein* attached to *HDL, VLDL* and *chylomicrons*. Apo E is cardioprotective and in a fasting state 70% of it is carried by HDL, but after a meal it attaches to triglyceride-rich VLDL and chylomicrons, removing them from circulation by binding them to specific cell types, thus decreasing *atherosclerosis*.
Genetic defects in apo E may result in familial dysbetalipoproteinaemia and are also associated with multiple sclerosis and Alzheimer's disease. Genetic defects in apoB100 and apoC2 also occur but are rare.

Apoptosis. Natural cell death mechanism.

Aspirin. Acetylsalicylic acid derived from the bark of willow trees that reduces blood viscosity and inflammation of body tissues.

ASHD. Atherosclerotic heart disease.

Arteriosclerosis. Hardening of the arteries caused by *atherosclerosis*.

Atheroma. Fatty deposits and atherosclerotic plaques in arteries.

Atherosclerosis. A disease begun in childhood involving formation of plaques of oxidized *cholesterol* that can cause blockage of arteries. The blood vessel wall beneath becomes *anoxic* and hardens (*arteriosclerosis*). Dislodged fragments from plaques can cause strokes or heart attack.

B6, B12. See *folic acid*.

Beta-carotene. Found mostly in carrots. One of several carotenoids primarily found in yellow, orange and red fruits and vegetables. An *antioxidant* which is metabolized in the body to produce vitamin A.

Blood pressure (BP). A measure of resistance to flow in the capillaries. As these are progressively clogged with *cholesterol* BP increases. High BP (hypertension) damages the circulatory system, leading to heart attack or stroke.

Body Mass Index (BMI) = weight (kg)/[height (m)]^2.
e.g., if you weigh 67 kg and are 1.88 m tall then your BMI = 19. Underweight: BMI <19. Normal: BMI 20-25. Overweight: BMI 25-30.

Bypass. Coronary artery bypass graft (CABG). Open heart surgery in which a leg vein or breast artery is grafted to connect the aorta to a coronary artery just beyond a *cholesterol* blockage.

Calcium. Needed for bones. Supplementation helps reduce osteoporosis, especially in women. *Magnesium* is important in the regulation of calcium and suggested intake is a third of that of calcium. One study showed that taking 1200 mg of calcium daily lowered BP 12% in men but other studies have not found this, perhaps because synergistic magnesium was not taken into account as well.

Carbohydrates. Starches and sugars in foods that are primarily used as a source of energy.

Cardiomyopathy. Chronic disease and thence weakening of the heart muscle, resulting in an enlarged heart.

CHD. Coronary heart disease. Also **CVD** = cardiovascular disease.

Chelation. Bonding of a metallic atoms to organic molecules. Used to treat heavy metal poisoning and to treat *atherosclerosis*.

Cholesterol. White waxy substance produced by the liver. Small amounts form part of the cell membranes. Absorbs *triglycerides* to form *lipoproteins* that circulate with the blood. Made by the body and found in meat, egg yolk, milk and cheese. Excess causes *atherosclerosis*.

Cholestin-3. Food supplement derived from Hong Qu, a *cholesterol* inhibiting yeast from rice fermentation.

Chylomicron. A large *lipoprotein* produced in the intestines which, along with *VLDL*, is largely responsible for carrying *triglycerides*. Chylomicrons contain several types of apolipoproteins, including apoA1 and apoB48, but not apoB100. As apoB48 is not recognized by LDL receptors chylomicron remnants are largely cleared by the liver whereas LDL is free to provide *cholesterol* to peripheral tissues.

Coenzyme Q10 (CoQ10). An *antioxidant* available in supplement form often prescribed for patients who have suffered heart failure.

Coronary arteries. The arteries that carry blood through the heart.

Coronary calcification. The development of bone tissue in atherosclerotic coronary arteries.

C-reactive protein (CRP). Raised blood levels of this indicate inflammation in the body, perhaps clogged blood vessels when the result may be rupture of a plaque and release of a blood clot.

DHA. Docosahexaenoic acid, along with *EPA* one of two important *omega-3 fatty acids* found in fish oil.

DHEA. Dehydroepaindrosterone, a precursor to testosterone and oestrogen, which is protective against heart disease.

Diabetes. Polygenic disease characterized by high blood glucose levels.

DNA. Deoxyribonucleic acid. Along with *RNA* one of two nucleic acids found in all cells.

Endothelial-derived relaxation factor (EDRF). Nitric oxide (*NO*) which relaxes/expands blood vessels.

EDTA. Ethylenediamine tetraacetic acid. Used to treat heavy metal poisoning by *chelation* and chelate calcium from atherosclerotic arteries.

Electrocardiogram (ECG). Oscilloscope visualization of the electrical activity in heart muscle.

Ellagic acid. Polyphenol *antioxidant* which plants convert into ellagitannins, glucosides which regenerate ellagic acid when eaten.

Endothelium. Lining of blood and lymphatic vessels.

EPA. Eicosapentaenoic acid, along with *DHA* one of two important *omega-3 fatty acids* found in fish oil.

Essential nutrients. Not made in the body. Must be obtained from foods.

Familial combined hyperlipidemia (FCH), also called familial hyercholesterolemia. Commonest inherited *cholesterol* disorder with associated high risk of premature cardiac disease affecting one in 100 people. People with FCH may have high *LDL* and/or *triglyceride* levels.

Fibre. Insoluble fibre (roughage) is largely undigested and excreted but helps clean the intestinal walls and does not affect *cholesterol* levels. Water-soluble fibre absorbs bile acids laden with cholesterol in the intestines and is excreted, thus reducing blood cholesterol levels.

Flavonoids. Type of polyphenol found especially in highly coloured fruits and vegetables and also red wine.

Folic acid (folate). Found in several foods. Necessary for *homocysteine* metabolism. Homocysteine levels build up with age but can be corrected with folate, B6 and B12 supplementation. B6 should be adequate in the diet but can be boosted by the occasional multivitamin tablet. B12 is difficult to obtain without meat, especially offal, but can be obtained in multivitamin, B-complex or some folate tablets.

Free radical. Produced during processing of oxygen and can cause oxidation of *cholesterol*.

Garlic. Reduces *cholesterol* and *triglyceride* levels. Also reduces blood viscosity and promotes *antioxidant* activity.

HDL. High density *lipoprotein* or HDL-C is the 'good' *cholesterol* that lines the blood vessels and also takes unused *LDL* back to the liver before it can attach to artery walls. Main protein is *apoA1*.

HIV. Human immunodeficiency virus that causes AIDS.

Homocysteine is derived from methionine, an *amino acid* made in the body. It is also found in animal protein. High blood levels increase *atherosclerosis*.

HPV. Human papilloma virus.

HRT. Hormone replacement therapy (for menopause).

Hypoganodism. Deficient activity of testis or ovary.

L-arginine. An essential *amino acid*. The body manufactures some of our L-arginine needs but additional supplies are also needed from protein foods, the healthiest choices being dried beans, legumes, peas, fish, soy, nonfat milk and nuts.

LDL. Low density *lipoprotein*. Contains *apoB100* and carries *cholesterol* manufactured by the liver to the body cells. LDL cholesterol or LDL-C, particularly the *Lp(a)* form, is the 'bad' cholesterol that causes plaques.

LDL pattern B. Substantial proportion of *LDL* is *small dense LDL*.

Lecithin-cholesterol acyltransferase (LCAT). Enzyme which esterifies free *cholesterol* for sequestration in the core of *HDL* and *LDL*. Important in *reverse cholesterol transport*. Also reduces the effects of oxidized LDL. Deficiency in LCAT may be genetic, causing a number of diseases.

Linseeds. The seed of flax. Rich in omega oils and used with lecithin in the "Mohr Formula' for atherosclerosis (see ch. 2).

Limonene. Aromatic substance derived from orange peels and found in a number of essential oils, for example Idaho balsam fir. Has been found effective in killing cancer cells and in cancer treatment.

Lipoprotein. Hydrophobic core of *cholesterol* esters, *triglycerides*, fatty acids, and fat-soluble vitamins with a hydrophilic layer of *apolipoproteins*, *phospholipids* and *cholesterol*. Lipoproteins circulate in the bloodstream to maintain the *endothelium* that lines blood and lymphatic vessels, and the epithelial layers covering the organs and the cell membranes.

Lipoprotein (a) or Lp(a). *LDL* particle manufactured in the liver with proteins *apo(a)* and *apo B100* attached. Lp(a) is used for arterial repair and elevated levels are an indicator for *atherosclerosis*.

Lycopene. A type of carotenoid and *antioxidant* found especially in tomatoes that apparently retards or reverses aging of cells in the prostrate gland that promote cancer.

Lysine. Amino acid important in collagen formation and used in the Pauling Therapy (see ch. 2).

Macrophage. Large phagocytic (capable of absorbing foreign matter) white blood cell (leucocyte) usually found at points of infection.

Magnesium. Mineral essential for nerve impulses, muscle action, energy metabolism and cellular energy storage. Known to lower *BP*, dilate arteries and normalize heart rhythms after heart attack.

Melanoma. Malignant neoplasm of the skin involving melanocytes, cells in the basal skin layer that produce melanin.

Minoxidil. Proprietary compound used as a vasodilator and also in hair growth formulas to treat baldness.

Monounsaturated fats. Found in canola, olive and peanut oil. If substituted for *saturated fats TC* level may fall and *HDL* level may rise.

MSG. Monosodium glutamate, a widely used food additive.

Nicotinic acid (niacin). Acidic form of vitamin B3. Reduces *cholesterol* and *triglyceride* levels and stimulates formation of *prostaglandins*. Dilates blood vessels and can cause flushing of skin and headaches.

Nicotinamide (niacinamide). Formed by acid-base chemical reaction of *nicotinic acid* in the liver. 500 mg tablets may be equivalent to about 100 mg of nicotinic acid. Taken over months (rather than weeks) this will contribute to *cholesterol* reduction as part of a comprehensive diet and supplements program. Does not cause flushing.

NO. Chemical formula for nitric oxide, the *endothelial-derived relaxation factor* (EDRF).

Occlusion. Closure or blockage (of a blood vessel).

Omega-3 and omega-6 fatty acids. Two types of 'essential' fatty acids which lower *cholesterol* and *triglyceride* levels and reduce blood viscosity.

ORAC. Oxygen Radical Absorbance Capacity. A measure of the oxygen radical absorption capacity of foods estimated by ferric reducing power and expressed as micromole Trolox equivalent per 100 grams (microTE/100 gm). The ORAC test is accurate to +/- 5%.

Osteoporosis. Loss of bone tissue resulting in fragile porous bones attributable to a lack of calcium and common in postmenopausal women.

Pancreatic enzymes. Used in the amygdalin (vitamin B17) Metabolic Therapy. These help 'unmask' the malignant cells, making it easier to destroy them.

Pectin. Water soluble fibre found in fruits and vegetables. May help tackle atherosclerosis and cancer.

Percent Atheroma Volume (PAV). $PAV = 100(A_{int} - L)/A_{int}$ with $A_{int} =$ internal cross sectional area (CSA) of artery and L = CSA of lumen.

Peroxidase. An enzyme that catalyzes the oxidation of various substances by peroxides.

PGI$_2$. *Prostacyclin.*

Phospholipid or **phosphatide.** Fat-like organic compound containing phosphate. The phospholipids, with the sphingolipids, the glycolipids, and the *lipoproteins*, are called complex lipids.

Phytosterols (sterols). Plant substances similar to *cholesterol* that compete with *cholesterol* for intestinal absorption and thus reduce cholesterol absorption.

Policosanol. A mixture of sugar cane wax alcohols which is claimed to improve *cholesterol* levels in 85% of patients in 8 weeks.

Polyunsaturated fats. Found in corn, safflower and sunflower oils. If substituted for *saturated fats* both *TC* and *HDL* levels may fall. Some studies have linked to colon cancer.

Procyanidins. Powerful *antioxidant* polyphenol compounds found particularly in cocoa and some red wines.

Prostacyclin or **PGI$_2$.** A prostaglandin stimulated by niacin and fish oil supplementation.

Prostaglandins. Chemicals that perform many functions including maintaining healthy blood vessels.

Proteins. The essential building blocks containing *amino acids*, carbon, hydrogen and oxygen.

PSA, prostate-specific antigen. An enzyme produced by both benign and malignant prostate cells. Elevated PSA levels are used to diagnose prostate cancer and to test the efficacy of treatment.

Punicalagins. Tannins, large polyphenol compounds found in pomegranates and only a few shrubs and flowering trees. Mainly responsible for the potent *antioxidant* effects and health benefits of pomegranate which seems to have an optimal mix of polyphenols.
Eight ounces of pomegranate juice contains 280 - 375 mg of punicalagins.

PVD. Peripheral vascular disease.

Quercetin. A powerful *antioxidant* found in red wine, onions (particularly red ones), broccoli and tea.

Quinones. A class of cyclic organic compounds which occur as biological pigments in plants. The K vitamins are *napthoquinones*.

RDI. Recommended daily intake.
Also **RDA**, recommended daily allowance.

Receptors. Molecules on the cells which are the attachment points of apolipoproteins carried by lipoproteins which, once attached, deliver *cholesterol* and *triglycerides* to the cells. Other receptors also anchor other proteins such as tumour suppressor proteins p53, p16 and p21 and tumour suppressor genes such as the *retinoblastoma gene*.

Regression. Shrinkage of plaques which tends to occur with *LDL* < 100. Also shrinkage of tumours.

Resistance training. Exercises such as weightlifting, sometimes aimed primarily at building muscles.

Reverse cholesterol transport (RCT). Lipid-poor, nascent, discoidal HDL/apoA1 absorb *cholesterol* from the *triglyceride*-rich *lipoproteins VLDL* and *chylomicrons*, and to a small extent from plaque *macrophages*. The then mature, spheroidal *HDL* transport it to the liver for excretion.

RNA. Ribonucleic acid. With *DNA* a building block for cells.

RPR. Resting pulse rate.

Saturated fat. Found in red meat, white meat fat, milk, butter, cheese, and coconut & palm oils. Increases *cholesterol* levels.

Saw palmetto. Herb used to treat *benign prostate hypertrophy*.

Selenium. 34th in the periodic table of the elements. Arsenic, once prescribed in minute dosages in homeopathy, is 33rd.

Small dense LDL (SDL). A particularly dangerous form of *LDL*.

Stasis. Stoppage of flow of blood or urine.

Statins. Introduced in the 1980s, statins are the most effective *cholesterol* lowering medications. They lower *LDL* levels by up to 30 - 40% but, until recently, are less effective in raising *HDL* levels.

Stenosis. Constricted or decreased in diameter.

Target heart rate. The heart rate during *aerobic exercise* that strengthens heart muscle.

Tocotrienols. See vitamin E.

TIA. Transient Ischemic Attack or mild stroke.

Total cholesterol (TC) = *HDL* + *LDL* + *VLDL*.
where VLDL = (*Triglycerides* / 5) approximately.

Trans fat. Created by hydrogenation of canola, corn, olive and sunflower oils. Similar effects to *saturated fat*. Found in fast foods.

Triglycerides. Fat carried in the bloodstream by *chylomicrons*, a large *lipoprotein* produced in the intestines, and by *VLDL* which is produced in the liver. *LDL* also carries a small amount of *triglycerides*.

Variant angina. Heart pains brought on by mental stress – see the section *Magnesium for Prinzmetal's Variant Angina* in Chapter 13.

Vitamin C (L-ascorbic acid). An *antioxidant* water-soluble vitamin.

Vitamin E. Usually in the form dl-alpha-Tocopheryl-acetate or dl-alpha-Tocopheryl-succinate - the 'dl' denoting the synthetic form, whereas 'd' denotes the (preferable/superior) natural form.
An *antioxidant* fat-soluble vitamin.
The tocotrienol forms of vitamin E are more powerful *antioxidants*. Rice bran is a good source, others being barley, cocoa butter, coconut oil, and wheat germ.
The safest course is to take full spectrum vitamin E, that is, containing tocotrienols as well as tocopherols.

Vitamin K. Needed for blood clotting. Vitamin K_1 is found in green, leafy vegetables. Vitamin K_2 is made by bacteria in the large intestine and is the important form in mammalian tissue.

VLDL. Very low density *lipoprotein*. Contains several types of *apolipoproteins*, including *apoB100, apoC* and *apoE*. Larger *lipoprotein* especially likely to cause strokes and other vascular problems.

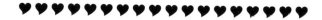

Glossary

REFERENCES

Note: details for some periodical articles are given in parentheses in the text.

Alderman et al., Ten-year follow-up of survival and myocardial infarction in the Randomized Coronary Artery Study. *Circulation* 82 (1990) 1629.

Armstrong MC et al., Regression of Coronary Atherosclerosis in Rhesus Monkeys. *Circulation Research* 27 (1970) 59.

Atkins RC, *Dr Atkins' Diet Revolution.* Bantam, New York 1973.

Atkins RC, *Dr Atkins' Super-Energy Diet.* Bantam, New York 1978.

Atrens D, Curthoys I, *The Neurosciences and Behaviour,* 2nd edn. Academic Press, Sydney 1982.

Aviram M, Rosenblat M, Gaitini D, et al., Pomegranate juice consumption for 3 years by patients with carotid artery stenosis reduces common carotid intima-media thickness, blood pressure and LDL oxidation. *Clin Nutr.* 23/3 (2004) 423-33.

Benderly M, Boyko V, Goldbourt U, Apolipoproteins and Long-Term Prognosis in Coronary Heart Disease Patients. *American Heart Journal* 157/1 (2009) 103-110.

Berg K, Mohr J, Genetics of the Lp System. *Acta Genet.* 13(4) (1963) 349-360.

Biehler RF, *Child Development, An Introduction.* Houghton Mifflin, Boston MA 1981.

Bingham J, Hadfield J, *The New Runner, Running and Walking for Fitness, Weight Loss and Fun,* Rodale, London, 2007.

Blankenhorn DH, Hodis HN, Atherosclerosis--reversal with therapy. *The Western Journal of Medicine* 159/2 (1993) 172-9.

Blumenfeld A, *Heart Attack: Are You a Candidate?* Paul S Eriksson Inc., New York 1964.

Bock K, Sabin N, *The Road to Immunity, How to Survive and Thrive in a Toxic World,* Pocket Books, New York, 1997.

Borushek A, *Allan Borushek's Calorie, Fat & Carbohydrate Counter,* Hinkler Books, Melbourne, 2014.

REFERENCES

Borushek A, Borushek J, *The Complete Australian Heart Disease Prevention Manual.* Family Health Publications, Perth, 1981.

Brookes-Simpkins R, *Improve Your Eyes at Home.* L.N. Fowler, London 1968.

Brown L, Rosner B, Willett WW, Sacks FM. Cholesterol-lowering effects of dietary fiber: a meta-analysis. *Am J Clin Nutr* 69/1 (1999) 30-42.

Buchman AL, Dubin M, Jenden D et al., Lecithin increases plasma free choline and decreases hepatic steatosis in long-term total parenteral nutrition patients. *Gastroenterol* 102(4) (1992) 1363-1370.

Brook JG, Linn S, Aviram M, Dietary soya lecithin decreases plasma triglyceride levels and inhibits collagen- and ADP-induced platelet aggregation. *Biochem Med Metab Biol* 35 (1986) 31-39.

Byers SO, Friedman M, Effect of infusion of phosphatides upon atherosclerotic aorta in situ and as an ocular aortic implant. *Journal of Lipid Research* 1 (1960) 343-348.

Canner PL, Berge KG, Wenger NK, Stamler J, Friedman L, Prineas RJ & Freidewald W, Fifteen year mortality Coronary Drug Project; patients long term benefit with niacin. *American Coll Cardiology* 8 (1986) 1245-1255.

Carlson LA et al., Pronounced lowering of serum levels of lipoprotein Lp(a) in hyperlipidemic subjects treated with nicotinic acid. *Archives Int. Med.* 226 (1989) 271.

Carper, Jean, *The Miracle Heart - The Ultimate Guide to Preventing and Curing Heart Disease by Diet and Supplements.* Harper, New York, 2000.

Carr, Allen, *Allen Carr's Easy Way to Stop Smoking,* 3rd edn. Penguin, London, 1999.

Cartmel B, Moon TE, Levine N, Effects of long-term intake of retinol on selected clinical and laboratory indexes. *Am J Clin Nutr* 69 (1999) 937-43.

Cheraskin E, Ringsdorf WM Jr, Brecher A, *Psychodietetics: Food As the Key to Emotional Health.* Stein & Day, New York, 1974.

Cheraskin E, Ringsdord WM, Clark JW, *Diet and Disease.* Rodale Press, Emmaus Pa, 1975.

Christensen A, *Heart Health: An American Yoga Association Wellness Guide.* Twin Streams Books, New York, 2001.

Clements FW, Rogers JF, *You and Your Food, Diet and Nutrition for Australians and New Zealanders.* AH & AW Reed, Sydney, 1967.

Clarke, HH, *Application of Measurement to Health and Physical Education,* 4th edn. Prentice-Hall, Englewood Cliffs NJ, 1967.

REFERENCES

Consumer Guide, *The Vitamin Book.* Fireside, New York, 1979.

Cooke JP (with J Zimmer), *The Cardiovascular Cure.* Broadway Books, New York, 2002.

Cooper K, *Advanced Nutritional Therapies.* Nelson, Nashville, 1996.

Corder R, *The Red Wine Diet.* Sphere, London, 2007.

Corrao G, Bagnardi V, Zambon A, Exploring the dose-response relationship between alcohol consumption and the risk of several alcohol-related conditions: a meta-analysis. *Addiction* 94 (1999) 1551-73.

Council on Scientific Affairs, Dietary and Pharmacological Therapy for the Lipid Risk Factors. *JAMA* 250 (1983) 1873.

Creswell A, Drug in stroke alert. *The Australian,* October 19, 2005.

Creswell A, Cholesterol mutation in spotlight, *The Weekend Australian,* September 6-7, 2008.

Dalessandri KM, Reduction of lipoprotein(A) in postmenopausal women [letter]. *Arch Intern Med* 161 (2001)772-3.

Davis A, *Let's Get Well.* New American Library, NY, 1972.

Donatelle RJ, *Health, The BASICS green edition,* Pearson Benjamin Cummings, San Francisco CA, 2011.

Duguid JB, Thrombosis as a factor In the pathogenesis of coronary atherosclerosis. *J Pathol Bacteriol* 58 (1946) 207-212.

Dreon DM, Vranizan, Krauss RM, Austin MA, Wood PD, The effects of polyunsaturated fat vs. monounsaturated fat on plasma lipoproteins. *JAMA* 263 (1990) 2462.

Eady J, *Additive Elert,* Additive Alert P/L, Mullalo WA , 2006.

Eliaz I, Hotchkiss AT, Fishman ML, Rode D, The effect of modified citrus pectin on urinary excretion of toxic elements. *Phytother Res* 20/10 (2006) 859-864.

Ellis R, *A Short History of the Nutritional Approach to the Prevention and Cure of Cardiovascular Disease.* Essay posted on website saveyourheart.com, 2005.

Enstrom JE, Kanim LE, Klein MA, Vitamin C intake and mortality among a sample of the United States population. *Epidemiology* 3/3 (1992) 194-202.

Entwistle IR, *Exacta Medical Reference Tables and Data.* Picturettes Ltd, Liverpool, circa 1965.

European Heart Journal: article on a German study of suppression of FMD effect of black tea by milk. Quoted in *The Australian,* 'Milking tea of its goodness,' 10/1/2006.

REFERENCES

Expert Panel on Detection, Evaluation and Treatment of High Blood Cholesterol in Adults. Executive Summary of the third report of the National Cholesterol Education Program (NCEP) expert panel on detection, evaluation, and treatment of high blood cholesterol in adults (Adult Treatment Panel III). *JAMA* 285 (2001) 2486-2497.

Eyton A, *The F-Plan Calorie and Fibre Chart.* Penguin, Melbourne, 1982.

Family Medical, *Men's Health.* Geddes and Grosset, New Lanark, Scotland, 2000.

Firshein R, *The Neutraceutical Revolution,* Riverhead Books, New York, 1998.

Fischer WL, *Secrets to a Healthy Heart and Low Cholesterol.* Fischer Publishing Corporation, Canfield Ohio, 1993.

Fowkes FGR, Housely E, Macintyre CCA et al., Variability of ankle and brachial systolic pressures in the measurement of atherosclerotic peripheral arterial disease. *J Epidemiology & Community Health* 42 (1988) 128.

Friedman M, Homer R, Byers SG, An evaluation of potassium iodide as a therapeutic agent in the treatment of experimental hypercholesterolemia and atherosclerosis. *J Clinical Investigations* 35/9 (1956) 1015-1024.

Friedman M, Byers SO, Rosenman RH, Resolution of aortic atherosclerotic infiltrations in the rabbit by phosphatide infusion. *Proc Soc. Exp. Bio. Med.* 95 (1957) 586-588.

Fulder S, *The Garlic Book.* Avery, Garden City Park NY, 1997.

Galton D, *In Our Own Image, Eugenics and the Genetic Modification of People,* Little Brown, London, 2001.

Gardner H (ed.), *Health Policy, Development, Implementation, and Evaluation in Australia,* Churchill Livingstone, Melbourne (1992).

Gaziano JM, Buring JE, Breslow JL et al., Moderate alcohol intake, increased levels of high-density lipoprotein and its subfractions, and decreased risk of myocardial infarction. *New England J Medicine,* 329 (1993) 1829.

Geoly K, Diamond LH, Ascorbic acid and hypertriglyceridemia. *Ann. Int. Med.* 93 (1980) 551.

Gey et al., Inverse correlation between plasma vitamin E and mortality from ischemic heart disease in cross cultural epidemiology. *American Journal of Clinical Nutrition* 53 (January 1991): 326-334.

Gielen S, Schuler G, Hambrecht R, Exercise training in coronary artery disease and coronary vasomotion. *Circulation* 103 (2001) e1-e6.

Gillinov M, Nissen S, *Heart 411, The Only Guide to Heart Health You'll Ever Need,* Three Rivers Press, NY (2012).

Gittleman AL, *The Fast Track Detox Diet For Rapid Weight Loss, Improved Health and Vitality,* Century, London, 2005.

Gold, Lee, *Low Fat Foods Fast, 100 low-fat meals that beat the clock,* Pan MacMillan, Sydney, 2002.

Gonzalez-Gronow M, Edelberg JM, Pizzo SV, Further characterization of the cellular plasminogen binding site: evidence that plasminogen 2 and lipoprotein(A) compete for the same site. *Biochemistry* 28 (1989) 2374-2377.

Gottlieb W et al. (editors), *The Doctors Book of Home Remedies.* Bookman Press, Melbourne, 1990.

Gottlieb Bill, *Alternative Cures, The Most Effective Natural Home Remedies for 160 Health Problems,* Rodale, New York, 2000.

Griffith HW, Moore, SW, *Complete Guide to Prescription & Nonprescription Drugs,* Perigree, New York, 2013.

Hajjar KA et al., Lipoprotein(A) Modulation of endothelial cell surface fibrinolysis and its potential role in atherosclerosis. *Nature* 339 (1989) 303-305.

Haney D, Cleaning the pipes. *The Weekend Australian,* 7th Feb. 2005.

Harpel PC, Gordon BR, Parker TS, Plasminogen catalyzes binding of lipoprotein(A) to immobilized fibrinogen and fibrin, *Proc. Natl. Acad. Sci. USA* 86 (1989) 3847-3851.

Haynes SG, Feinleib M, Kannel WB, The relationship of psychological factors to coronary heart disease. *Am J Epidemiology* 37 (1980) 111.

Heber D, *Natural Remedies for a Health Heart.* Avery, New York, 1998.

Hegele RA, Is regression of coronary atherosclerosis possible by infusing recombinant apolipoprotein A-I? *CMAJ* 170/6 (2004).

Hodis HN, Mack WJ, LaBree L, Cashin-Hemphill L, Sevanian A, Johnson R, Azen SP, Serial coronary angioplastic evidence that antioxidant vitamin intake reduces progression of coronary artery atherosclerosis. *JAMA* 272 (1995) 1845.

Holford P, Colson D, *Optimum Nutrition for Your Child,* Piatkus, London, 2008.

Holford C, *New Optimum Nutrition For The Mind,* Basic Health, Laguna Beach CA, 2009.

Horsey J, Livesley B, Dickerston JWT, Ischaemic heart disease and aged patients: effects of ascorbic acid on lipoproteins, *Journal of Human Nutrition,* 35 (1981) 53-58.

REFERENCES

Howlader ZH, Kamiyama S, Murakami Y, Ito M, Komai M, Furukawa Y, Lecithin Cholesterol Acyltransferase reduces the adverse effects of oxidized low-density lipoprotein while incurring damage itself. *Bioscience, Biotechnology, and Biochemistry* 65/11 (2001) 2496-2503.

Hsu HY, Nicholson AC, Pomerantz KB, Kaner RJ, Hajjar DP, Altered cholesterol trafficking in herpes virus-infected arterial cells. Evidence for viral protein kinase-mediated cholesterol accumulation. *J Biol Chem* 270/33 (August 1995) 19630-7.

Jackson CL, Dreaden TM, Theobald LK, Tran NM, Beal TL, Eid M, Yun Gao M, Shirley RB, Stoffel MT, Kumar MV, Mohnen D, Pectin induces apoptosis in human prostate cancer cells: correlation of apoptotic function with pectin structure. *Glycobiology* 17/August (2007) 805-819.

Jacobsen DW, Homocysteine and vitamins in cardiovascular disease. *Clinical Chemistry* 44 (1998) 1833-1843.

Jacques PF, Hartz SC, McGandy RB, Jacob RA, Russell RM, Ascorbic acid, HDL, and total plasma cholesterol in the elderly. *J Am Coll Nutr* 6/2 (April 1987)169-74.

Jelinek G, *Overcoming Multiple Sclerosis, An Evidence-Based Guide to Recovery,* Allen & Unwin, Sydney (2010).

Jimenez MA, Scarino ML, Vignolini F, Mengheri E, Evidence that polyunsaturated lecithin induces a reduction in plasma cholesterol level and favorable changes in lipoprotein composition in hypercholesterolemic rats. *J. Nutr.* 120/7 (July 1990) 659-67.

Jochems R, *Dr Moerman's Anti-Cancer Diet.* Avery, New York, 1990.

Johnson T, Pomegranate, powerful protection for aging arteries - and much more. *Life Extension Foundation Journal* May 2007, 55-62.

Kalb R, Holland N, Giesser B, *Multiple Sclerosis for Dummies,* Wiley, Indianopolis, 2007.

Kamanna VS, Kashyap ML, Mechamism of action of niacin. *Am J Cardiol.* 101/8A (2008) 20B-26B.

Karin KM, Park JJ, Postle J, Cottrill A, Ward MR, Frequency of late drug-eluting stent thrombosis with non-cardiac surgery. *The American Journal of Cardiology,* www.ajconline.org 2010).

Kiat H, *EastWest Medical Makeover: 14 days to feeling fabulous.* Image of Distinction P/L, Sydney, 2002.

Key TJ, Fraser GE, Thorogood M, Appleby PN, Beral V, Reeves G, Burr ML, Chang-Claude J, Frentzl-Bayme R, Kuzma JW, Mann J, McPherson K, Mortality in vegetarians and non-vegetarians: detailed findings from a collaborative analysis of 5 prospective studies. *Am J Clinical Nutrition* 70 (1999) 516S - 524S.

Kim I, Williamson DF, Byers T, Koplan JP, Vitamin supplement use and mortality. *Am J Public Health* 84/6 (1994) 1035-7.

Ko AH, Dollinger MD, Rosenbaum MD, *Everyone's Guide to Cancer Therapy* 5th edn, Andrews McNeels Publishing, Kansas City, Missouri, 2008.

Kohlmeir L, Kark JD, Gomez-Garcia E, Martin BC, Steck SE, Kardinaal AFM, Ringstad J, Thamm M, Masaev V, Riemensma R, Martin-Moreno JM, Huttunen JK, Kok FJ, Lycopene and myocardial infarction risk in the Euramic study. *Am J Epidemiology* 146 (1997) 618.

Kowalski RE, *The 8-Week Cholesterol Cure,* Schwartz, Sydney, 1987.

Kowalski RE, *Take The Pressure Off Your Heart: 8 Weeks to Lower Blood Pressure Without Prescription Drugs.* New Holland, Sydney, 2006.

Krumdieck C, Butterworth CE Jr, Ascorbate-Cholesterol-Lecithin Interactions: factors of potential importance in the pathogenesis of atherosclerosis. *American Journal of Clinical Nutrition*, 27 (1974) 866-876, August.

Kurzweil R, *The 10% Solution for a Healthy Life, How to Eliminate Virtually All Risk of Heart Disease and Cancer.* Bookman Press, Melbourne, 1993.

Lapenna D, de Gioia S, Ciofani G, Mezzetti A, Ucchino S, Calafiore AM, Napolitano AM, Di Ilio C, Cuccurulo F, Glutathione-related antioxidant defenses in human atherosclerotic plaques. *Circulation* 97 (1998) 1930-4.

Lee WH, Lee L, *Concentrated Youth Restoring Foods*, m2m Direct/Bookman, Melbourne, 1994.

LeGro W, ed., *High-Speed Healing, The Fastest, Safest and Most Effective Shortcuts to Lasting Relief,* Rodale Press, Emmaus PA, 1991.

Leinweber C et al, *J Epidemiology Community Health,* 2009, doi:10.1136/jech.2009.088880.

Lemole MD, Gerald M, *The Healing Diet: A Total Health Program to Purify Your Lymph System and Reduce the Risk of Heart Disease.* William Morrow & Company, New York, 2000.

Leonard JN, Hofer JL, Pritikin N, *Live Longer Now, The First One Hundred Years of Your Life.* Grosset & Dunlap, New York, 1974.

Lewis GF, Rader DJ, New insights Into the regulation of HDL metabolism and reverse cholesterol transport. *Circulation Research* 96 (2005)1221-1232.

Lieberman S, Bruning N, *The Real Vitamin & Mineral Book,* 2nd edn. Avery, New York, 1997.

REFERENCES

Lonn E, Bosch J, Yusuf S, Sheridan P, Pogue J, Arnold JM, et al., HOPE and HOPE-TOO Trial Investigators. Effects of long-term vitamin E supplementation on cardiovascular events and cancer: a randomized controlled trial. *JAMA* 293 (2005)1338-47.

Lourie B, Smith R, *Toxin Toxout, Getting Harmful Chemicals Out of Our Bodies and Our World,* Univ. of Queensland Press, St Lucia QLD, 2013.

Lubkin IM, Larsen PD, *Chronic Illness, Impact and Interventions,* 6th edn, Jones & Bartlett, Sudbury MA, 2006.

Luckman J, Sorenson KC, *Medical-Surgical Nursing,* 2nd edn. Saunders WB, Philadelphia, 1980.

Maegraith D, Diabetics warned on vascular disease. *The Weekend Australian*, Jan. 24-25 2005.

Marchese R, Hill A, *The Essential Guide to Fitness for the fitness instructor,* Pearson/Prentice-Hall, Sydney, 2005.

Marcus BA, Hamps JS, Fisher ED, *How to Quit Smoking Without Gaining Weight.* American Lung Assocation/Rocket Books, New York, 2004.

Markus RA, Mack WJ, Azen SP, Hodis HN, Influence of lifestyle modification on atherosclerotic progression determined by ultrasonic change in the common carotid intima-media thickness. *American J Clinical Nutrition* 65 (1997) 1000.

Martin MJ et al., article in *The Lancet* 11 (1986) 933-936. Cited in World Book Multimedia Encyclopedia 1999.

Masharani U, *Diabetes Demystified, A Self-Teaching Guide,* McGraw-Hill, New York, 2007.

Mattson FH et al., Optimizing the effects of plant sterols on cholesterol absorption in man. *Am J Clinical Nutrition* 35 (1982) 697.

Mayo Clinic, *Mayo Clinic Heart Book.* William Morrow, New York, 2000.

McGowan MP, *Heart Fitness for Life.* Oxford University Press, New York, 1998.

Medeiros RW, *Chemistry, An Interdisciplinary Approach.* Van Nostrand Reinhold, New York, 1971.

Merrill S (ed.). *Medicines – More Than 3000 Drugs – What They Are and How They Work,* Bloomsbury, London, 1995.

Minirth F, Meier P, *Happiness is a Choice, The Symptoms, Causes, and Cures of Depression,* Baker Books, Grand Rapids, Michigan, 2007.

Mohr GA, A doubly curved isoparametric triangular shell element, *Computers & Structures* vol. 14, p 9 (1981).

Mohr GA, Application of penalty factors to a doubly curved quadratic shell element, *Computers & Structures* vol. 14, p 15 (1981).

Mohr GA, A finite element lubrication model. *Proc. 4th Australian Int. Conf. Finite Element Methods*, Melbourne University 1982.

Mohr GA, *Finite Elements for Solids, Fluids, and Optimization.* Oxford University Press, Oxford 1992.

Mohr GA, Finite element modeling and optimization of traffic flow networks, *Transportmetrica* 1 (2005) 151.

Mohr GA, *The Doomsday Calculation,* Xlibris, Sydney, 2012.

Mohr GA, *Curing Cancer & Heart Disease, Proven Ways to Combat Aging, Atherosclerosis & Cancer,* Xlibris, Sydney, 2012b.

Mohr GA, *Heart Disease, Cancer & Aging, Proven Neutraceutical & Lifestyle Solutions,* Horizon, Sydney, 2013.

Mohr GA, *Elementary Thinking for the 20th Century,* Xlibris, Sydney, 2014.

Mohr, GA, *The 8-Week+ Program to Reverse Cardiovascular Disease,* Book Venture, Ishpeming MI (2015).

Mohr GA, Sinclair R, Fear E, *Human Intelligence, Learning & Behaviour,* Inspiring Publishers, Canberra, 2017.

Morgan WJ, Meier KV (eds), *Philosophic Enquiry into Sport.* Human Kinetic Publishers Inc., Champaign IL, 1988.

Morton IKM, Hall JM, *Medicines, The Comprehensive Guide,* Bloomsbury, London, 1996.

Mosby Year Book Inc., *Mosbys Medical Encyclopedia,* London, 1995.

Mosley, Michael, *Should I Eat Meat,* BBC documentary program shown on Australia's SBS1 TV channel 7:30 PM, 1 June 2015.

Multiple Risk Factor Intervention Trial Research Group, Multiple Risk Factor Trial, risk factor changes and mortality. *JAMA* 248 (1982) 1465.

Murray F, *Program Your Heart for Health.* Larchmont Books, New York, 1977.

Murrell M, Khachigian LM, Ward MR, Divergent roles of NF-B and Egr-1 in flow-dependent restenosis after angioplasty and stenting. *Atherosclerosis* 214(2011) 65-72.

Myllyla R, Kuutti-Savolilanin ER, and Kivirikko KI, The role of ascorbate in the prolyl-hydroxylase reaction. *Biochem. Biophys. Res. Commun.* 83 (1978) 441-448.

Newcombe J (with L Writer), *No-one's Indestructible.* Pan MacMillan, Sydney, 2005.

Newman WP III, Wattingey W, Berenson GS, Autopsy studies in U.S. children and adolescents. Relationship of risk factors to atherosclerotic lesions. *Annals of NY Academy of Sciences*, 623 (1991) 16.

News-Medical.Net, *Nutritional supplement policosanol does not lower cholesterol levels.* 23/5/2006.

NHMRC (National Health and Medical Research Council), *Nutrient Reference Values,* nhc.nhmrc@nhmrc.gov.au, 2009.

NHMRC, *Australian Guidelines: To Reduce Health Risks from Drinking Alcohol.* NHMRC, Canberra, 2009.

Nicholls SJ et al., Statins, high-density lipoprotein cholesterol, and regression of coronary atherosclerosis. *JAMA* 297 (2007) 499-508.

Nissen SE, Tsunoda T, Tuzcu EM, Schoenhagen P, Cooper CJ, Yasin M, et al., Effect of recombinant ApoA-I Milano on coronary atherosclerosis in patients with acute coronary syndromes: a randomized controlled trial. *JAMA* 290/17 (2003) 2292-300.

Nissen SE, Nicholls SJ, Sipahi I, Libby P, Raichlen JS, Ballantyne CM, Davignon J, Erbel R, Fruchart JC, Tardif JC, Schoenhagen P, Crowe T, Cain V, Wolski K, Goormastic M, Tuzcu EM, Effect of very high-intensive statins therapy on regression of coronary atherosclerosis. *JAMA* 295 (2006) - published online March 13, 2006.

Nordoy A et al., Individual effects of saturated fatty acids and fish oil on plasma lipids and lipoproteins in normal men. *Am. J Clinical Nutrition* 57 (1993) 634.

Normand A, *The 10 Commandments of Losing Weight,* Penguin, Melbourne (2005).

Ogden J, *Health Psychology, A Textbook,* 4th edn, Open University Press/McGraw-Hill, Maidenhead, Berkshire, 2007.

Ohashi R, Mu H, Wang X, Yao Q, Chen C, Reverse cholesterol transport and cholesterol efflux in atherosclerosis. *QJM* 9812 (2005):845-856.

Ornish D, *Eat More, Weigh Less.* Bookman Press, Melbourne, 1993.

Ornish D, *Dr Dean Ornish's Program for Reversing Heart Disease.* Ivy Books/Ballantine, New York, 1996.

Ornish D, Brown D, Scherwitz LW et al., Can Lifestyle changes reverse coronary heart disease? *Lancet* 336 (1990) 336.

Pancharumiti N, Lewis CA, Sauberlich HE, Perkins LL, Go RC, Alvarez JO, Macaluso N, Acton RT, Copland RB, Cousins AL, Plasma homocysteine, folate and vitamin B12 concentration and risk for early onset of coronary heart disease. *Am. J. Clinical Nutrition* 59 (1994) 940.

Pantuck AJ, Leppert JT, Zomorodian N, et al., Cancer Therapy: Clinical Phase II Study of pomegranate juice for men with rising prostate-specific antigen following surgery or radiation for prostate cancer. *Clin Cancer Res.* 12/13 (2006) 4018-26.

Passwater R, *Supernutrition.* The Dial Press, New York, 1975.

Penguin Books Ltd, *Physical Fitness, 5BX 11-minute-a-day plan for men, XBX 12-minute-a-day plan for women.* Penguin, Harmondsworth, 1964.

Pincock S, DNA reveals the best diet for you. *The Weekend Australian* May 17-18 2008.

Plant J, Tidey G, *Eating For Better Health, How Dieting Can Help You Prevent Many Common Health Problems,* Virgin/Random House, London, 2010.

Prevention Magazine (book by editors of), *LifeSpan-Plus: 900 Natural Techniques to Live Longer.* MJF Books, New York, 1991.

Pritikin N, *The Pritikin Diet Permanent Weight-Loss Manual.* Grosset & Dunlap, New York, 1981.

Rath M, Pauling L, Solution to the puzzle of human cardiovascular disease: its primary cause is ascorbate deficiency leading to the deposition of lipoprotein(A) and fibrinogen/fibrin in the vascular wall. *Journal of Orthomolecular Medicine* 6 (1991) 125-134.

Rath M, Pauling L, Apoprotein(a) is an adhesive protein. *Journal of Orthomolecular Medicine* 6 (1991) 139-143.

Rath M, *Cellular Health Series - Cancer.* MR Publishing, Santa Clara CA (2001). Available at http://www4.dr-rath-foundation.org/pdf-files/

Rath M, *Cellular Health Series - The Heart.* MR Publishing, Santa Clara CA (2001). Available at http://www4.dr-rath-foundation.org/pdf-files/

Rath M, Niedzwiecki A, Nutritional supplement program halts progression of early coronary atherosclerosis documented by ultrafast computed tomography. *Journal of Applied Nutrition* 48 (1996) 68-78.

Rimm EB, Stampfer MJ, Ascherio A, Giovannucci E, Colditz GA, Willet WC et al., Vitamin E consumption and the risk of coronary heart disease in men. *New England J Med.* 328 (1993) 1450.

Rimm EB, Willett Wc, Hu FB, Simpson L, Colditz GA, Manson JE, Hennekens C, Stampfer MJ, Folate and vitamin B6 from diet and supplements in relation to risk of coronary heart disease among women. *JAMA* 279 (1998) 359.

Roizen MF, *Real Age: Are You as Young as You Can Be?* Harper-Collins, New York, 2001.

REFERENCES

Roizen MF & Mehmet CO, *You, The Owner's Manual, An Insider's Guide to the Body That Will Make You Healthier and Younger,* Piatkus, London, 2005.

Rudin D, Felix D, *Omega 3 Oils.* Avery, Garden City Park NY, 1996.

Salonen EM et al., Lipoprotein(A) binds to fibronectin and has serine proteinase activity capable of cleaving it. *EMBO J* 8(13) (1989) 4035-4040.

Sargent M, *Drinking and Alcoholism in Australia, A Power Relations Theory.* Longman Cheshire, Melbourne, 1979.

Satake K et al., Effects of magnesium on prostacyclin synthesis and intracellular free calcium concentration in vascular cells. *Magnesium Research* 17/1 (2004).

Schauss A G, Nutrition and behaviour, *J App Nutr* 35 (1983) 30-35.

Schuler G, Hambrecht R, Schlierf G, Niebauer J, Hauer K, Neumann J, Hoberg E, Drinkmann A, Bacher F, Grunze M, Regular physical exercise and low-fat diet. Effects on progression of coronary artery disease. *Circulation* 86 (1992) 1-11.

Schute WE, Taub HJ, *Vitamin E for Ailing and Healthy Hearts.* Pyramid Books, New York, 1972.

Schmidt-Nielson K, *Animal Physiology, Adaptation and Environment,* 2nd edn, Cambridge University Press, Cambridge (1979).

Sdringola S, Loghin C, Boccalandro F, Gould KL, Mechanisms of progression and regression of coronary artery disease by PET related to treatment intensity and clinical events at long-term follow-up. *Journal of Nuclear Medicine* 47/1 (2006) 59-67.

Sears B (with B Lawren), *Enter the Zone: A Dietary Road Map.* Regan Books, New York, 1995.

Seddon JM et al., Elevated homocysteine levels may be a biomarker for increased risk of AMD. *American Journal of Opthalmology,* Jan. 2006.

Selhub J, Jacques PJ, Bostom AG, D'Agostino RB, Wilson PW, Belanger AJ, O'Leary DH, Wolf PA, Schaefer EJ, Rosenberg IH, Association between plasma homocysteine concentrations and carotid-artery stenosis. *New England J Medicine* 332 (1995) 286.

Sniderman AD, Furberg CD, Keech A, et al., Apolipoproteins versus lipids as indices of coronary risk and as targets for statin treatment. *Lancet* 361 (Mar 2003) 777-80.

Somer E, *The Origin Diet.* Owl Books, New York, 2001.

Sorensen KD, Luckmann J, *Basic Nursing, A Psychophysiologic Approach,* 2nd edn, WB Saunders, Philadelphia PA, 1986.

REFERENCES

Spittle CR, Atherosclerosis and vitamin C. *The Lancet* ii (1971) 1280-1281.

Stamler J, Dyer AR, Shekelle RB, Neaton J, Stamler R, Relationship of baseline risk factors to coronary risk factors and all cause mortality, and to longevity: findings for long-term follow-up of Chicago cohorts. *Cardiology* 82 (1993) 191.

Stampfer MJ, Hennekens CH, Manson JR, Colditz GA, Rosner B, Willet WC, Vitamin E consumption and the risk of coronary disease in women. *New England J Medicine* 328 (1993) 1444.

Stampfer MJ, Malinow RM, Can lowering homocysteine levels reduce cardiovascular risk? *New England J Med.* 332 (1995) 286.

Stanton R, *Food and You: A Commonsense Approach to Nutrition.* Holt Rinehart and Winston, Sydney, 1984.

Stanway A, *Taking the Rough with the Smooth, Dietary Fibre and Your Health: A Medical Breakthrough.* Pan, London, 1976.

Steele M, *The Warburton Programme for Dieting, Health & Fitness.* Methuen Haynes, Sydney, 1985.

Sterna F, Bernerb YN, Polyakc Z, Komarnitskya M, Selad B, Hoppe M, Drora Y, Homocysteine effect on protein degradation rates. *Clinical Biochemistry* 37 (2004) 1002-1009.

Stone I, *The Healing Factor, Vitamin C Against Disease.* Grosset & Dunlap, New York, 1972.

Sudy M (editor), *Personal Trainer Manual.* American Council on Exercise & Reebok University Press, San Diego, 1991.

Sumner MD, Elliott-Eller M, Weidner G, et al., Effects of pomegranate juice consumption on myocardial perfusion in patients with coronary heart disease. *Am J Cardiol.* 96/6 (2005) 810-4.

Superko HR, Krauss RM, Coronary artery disease regression: convincing evidence for the benefit of aggressive lipoprotein management. *Circulation* 90 (1994) 1056.

Superko HR, *Before The Heart Attacks.* Rodale Press, London, 2004.

Tanigawa H, Billheimer JT, Tohyama J, Fuki IV, Ng DS, Rothblat GH, Rader DJ, Lecithin cholesterol acyltransferase expression has minimal effects on macrophage reverse cholesterol transport in vivo. *Circulation* 120 (2009)160-169.

Taylor CB et al., Atherosclerotic lesions in Rhesus Monkeys. *Archives of Pathology*, 76 (1963) 404.

Tchoua U, Gillard BK, Pownall HJ, HDL superphospholipidation enhances key steps in reverse cholesterol transport. *Atherosclerosis*, 2009 Oct 12 (Epub ahead of print).

Tran ZV, Weltiman A, Glass GV et al., The effects of exercise on blood lipids and lipoproteins: a meta-analysis of studies. *Med. Sci. Sports Exercise* 15 (1983) 393.

Turner KB, Studies on the prevention of cholesterol atherosclerosis in rabbits: The effects of whole thyroid and potassium iodide. *J Experimental Medicine* 58 (1933) 115-125.

Turner KB, Bidwell EH, Further observations on the blood cholesterol of rabbits in relation to atherosclerosis. *J Experimental Medicine* 62 (1935) 721-732.

Turner N, *The Hormone Diet, A 3-Step Program to Help You Lose Weight, Gain Strength, and Live Younger Longer,* Rodale, London, 2010.

Verlangieri AJ, The Role of Vitamin C in Diabetic and Nondiabetic Atherosclerosis. Bulletin, Bureau of Pharm. Services. Univ. Miss. Vol. 21, 1985.

Verlangieri AJ, Bush MJ, Prevention and regression of primate induced atherosclerosis by d-alpha-tocopherol. *Journal of the American College of Nutrition*, Vol 11, Issue 2 (1992) 131-138.

von Schacky C, Angerer P, Kothny W, et al., The effect of dietary omega-3 fatty acids on coronary atherosclerosis. A randomized, double-blind, placebo-controlled trial. *Ann Intern Med* 130 (1999) 554–62.

Wagner RH, *Environment and Man,* 3rd edn. WW Norton, New York, 1978.

Warshafsky S et al., Effect of garlic on total serum cholesterol. *Annals Internal Medicine* 119 (1993) 599.

Watson KE, Abrolat ML, Malone LL, Hogg JM, Doherty T, Deltrano R, Demer LL, Active serum vitamin D levels are inversely correlated with coronary calcification. *Circulation* 96 (1997) 1755.

Whitaker J, *Reversing Heart Disease, A Vital Program To Help Prevent, Treat, And Eliminate Cardiac Problems Without Surgery.* Warner Books, New York, 2002.

Weiss ML, Mann AE, *Human Biology and Behaviour,* 2nd edn. Little Brown, Boston, 1978.

Westcott P, *Food Solutions Healthy Heart: Recipes & advice for a healthier heart.* Hamlyn, London, 2002.

Williams MH, *The Ergogenics Edge, Pushing The Limits of Sports Performance,* Human Kinetics, Champaign IL (1998).

Williams RJ, *Nutrition Against Disease.* Pitman, NY, (1971).

REFERENCES

Willis GC, An experimental study of the intimal ground substance in atherosclerosis. *Canadian Medical Association Journal* 69 (1953) 17-22.

Willis GC, Light AW, Gow WS, Serial arteriography in atherosclerosis, *Canadian Medical Association Journal* 71 (1954).

Willis GC, The reversibility of atherosclerosis. *Canadian Medical Association Journal* 77 (1957) 106-109.

Wilston et al., Soy lecithin reduces plasma lipoprotein cholesterol and early atherogenesis in hypercholesterolemic monkeys and hamsters: beyond linoleate. *Atherosclerosis* 140(1) (Sep 1998)147-53.

Yang SS, Cheng KT, Lin YS, Liu YW, Hou WC. Pectin hydroxamic acids exhibit antioxidant activities in vitro. *J Agric Fo od Chem* 52/13 (2004):4270-4273.

Yuan, SW, *Foundations of Fluid Mechanics.* Prentice-Hall, Englewood Cliffs NJ 1967.

REFERENCES

THE DIY CARDIOVASCULAR CURE

- ➤ Atherosclerosis explained.
- ➤ The Mohr Formula for heart disease
- ➤ A unified theory of heart disease
- ➤ Diet do's & don'ts and food additives to avoid.
- ➤ Losing weight.
- ➤ Exercise and stress reduction.
- ➤ Quitting smoking
- ➤ Alcohol in moderation.
- ➤ Detailed diet plans and analysis.
- ➤ Dietary supplements for heart disease.
- ➤ The initial 8-week program to reduce cholesterol levels.
- ➤ The 2-year program to reverse atherosclerosis
- ➤ Comprehensive coverage of recent research results.

"A must read for anyone seriously concerned about their health. I can recommend this book to people who would like to know how to get the most out of life and isn't that everyone?"
Patricia Rae Oakley, Naturopath, 'Geranium health.'
"I have read your treatise on heart disease.
It's genius. I am adopting it straight away." – unsolicited comment.

G.A. Mohr did his PhD in Churchill College, Cambridge.
He published 50 international papers & more than 20 books, including:
- ➤ *A Microcomputer Introduction to the Finite Element Method*
- ➤ *Finite Elements for Solids, Fluids, and Optimization*
- ➤ *Curing Cancer & Heart Disease*
- ➤ *Heart Disease, Cancer and Ageing*
- ➤ *The Pretentious Persuaders*
- ➤ *The War of the Sexes*
- ➤ *The Variant Virus*
- ➤ *The Doomsday Calculation*
- ➤ *2045: A Remote Town Survives Global Holocaust*
- ➤ *The History and Psychology of Human Conflicts*
- ➤ *Elementary Thinking for the 21st Century*
- ➤ *The 8 Week+ Cure for Cardiovascular Disease*
- ➤ *The Scientific MBA*

and co-authored with Richard Sinclair & Edwin Fear
(nom de plumes for R. S. Mohr and P. E. Mohr)
- ➤ *World Religions*
- ➤ *The Brainwashed*
- ➤ *World War 3*
- ➤ *Human Intelligence, Learning & Behaviour*
- ➤ *The Evolving Universe: Relativity, Redshift & Life from Space*
- ➤ *The Psychology of Hope*
- ➤ *New Theories of the Universe, Evolution, and Relativity*
- ➤ *The Population Explosion*

Made in the USA
Lexington, KY
04 June 2018